The Cancer Wellness Cookbook

"Fighting cancer with good nutrition need not be boring or unappetizing. The new edition of the Cancer Lifeline cookbook combines sound, research-based nutritional advice with delicious recipes and practical meal planning and preparation tips. Unlike many other cookbooks, it includes per serving nutritional breakdowns that are helpful to those who are watching their protein, fat, and carbohydrate intake. This book is a wonderful resource for anyone who wants to eat well and stay healthy."

—*Patricia L. Dawson, MD, PhD, FACS; Medical Director, Swedish Cancer Institute Breast Program, Seattle, WA; Medical Director, True Family Women's Cancer Center, Seattle, WA*

"*The Cancer Wellness Cookbook* is a helpful resource for patients and their caregivers. More than a cookbook, it gathers information about biological interactions that been shown to affect cancer cells, and how certain foods may increase the body's ability to fight disease and handle side effects from treatment. The recipes are designed to help encourage cancer patients to eat, with intriguing tastes and textures that can keep patients interested in food. The healthy focus is good for the entire family, and is a great direction for the after cancer lifestyle."

—*Rick Clarfeld, MD; Breast Surgeon, Overlake Medical Clinics Breast Surgery, Bellevue, WA*

"*The Cancer Wellness Cookbook* is an excellent resource that is current, concise, and informative. The tips to help minimize acute problems are relevant and the basic principles of healthy eating will aid in successful cancer survivorship. I applaud Cancer Lifeline, the authors, and many collaborators for creating a book that not only will help patients and families, but will serve as an excellent primer for health care professionals."

—*Eric Taylor, MD; Radiation Oncology, Evergreen Health, Kirkland, WA*

The Cancer Wellness
Cookbook

Smart Nutrition and Delicious Recipes
for People Living with Cancer

KIMBERLY MATHAI, MS, RD, CDE

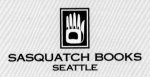

SASQUATCH BOOKS
SEATTLE

Printed in China
Published by Sasquatch Books
18 17 16 15 14   9 8 7 6 5 4 3 2 1

Editor: Gary Luke
Project editor: Nancy W. Cortelyou
Photographs: Olivia Brent
Design: Anna Goldstein
Food styling: Julie Hopper
Copy editor: Rachelle Longé McGhee

Library of Congress Cataloging-in-Publication Data is available.
ISBN: 978-1-57061-918-2
Sasquatch Books
1904 Third Avenue, Suite 710
Seattle, WA 98101
(206) 467-4300
www.sasquatchbooks.com
custserv@sasquatchbooks.com

DISCLAIMER: Cancer Lifeline makes no warranty of any nature, expressed
or implied, concerning the effectiveness of the recipes or diet suggestions included in this publication as a means to prevent or cure any form
of cancer.

---

*The Cancer Wellness Cookbook is available at a discount when purchasing in quan-
tity for sales promotions or corporate use. Special editions, including personalized
covers, excerpts, and corporate imprints, can be created when purchasing in large
quantities. For more information, please call Premium Sales at Random House at
(212) 572-2232 or email specialmarkets@randomhouse.com.*

DEDICATION

Cancer Lifeline and the author would like to thank all the cancer survivors—as well as their caregivers, family members, and friends—whose desire to make healthy nutritional choices, improve their sense of well-being, and take more control over their lives provided the inspiration for *The Cancer Wellness Cookbook.*

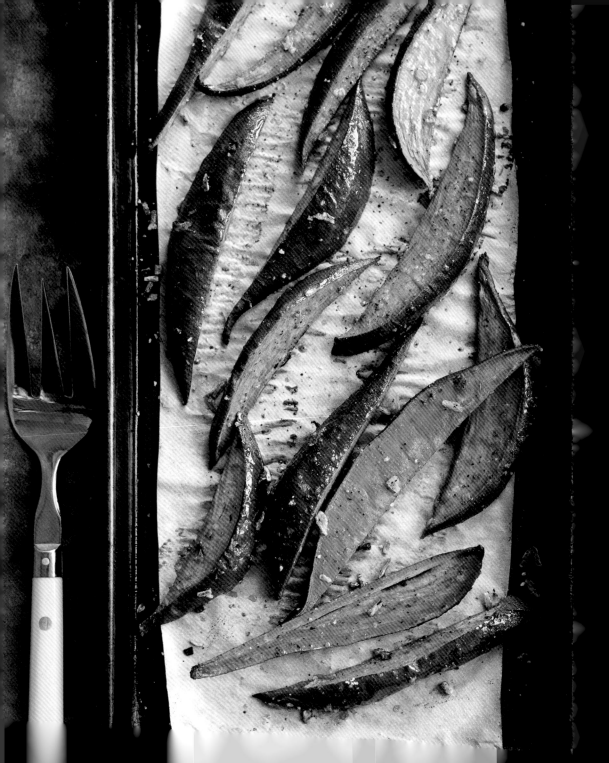

CONTENTS

RECIPE LIST

DESSERTS

INTRODUCTION

NEW SCIENCE CONTINUES TO EMERGE THAT LINKS CANCER SURVIVAL, risk of cancer recurrence, and cancer prevention with diet and physical activity. This scientific evidence is so compelling that the American Cancer Society estimates that nearly one-third of all cancer deaths are related to these two factors.

Nutrition can have a significant impact on preventing cancer and may also have a role in fighting cancer once it has developed. What's more, nutrition and other lifestyle factors may help lower cancer survivors' chances of developing secondary cancers and having recurrences.

Because good nutrition is so important before, during, and after treatment, *The Cancer Wellness Cookbook* is primarily for people living with cancer and for cancer survivors. However, this book is also intended for anyone interested in a health-conscious diet. It sets the stage for a healthier lifestyle from which we all can benefit.

The first edition of the cookbook, which was published in 1996, was created because clients of Cancer Lifeline kept asking, "So what do I eat now?" Cancer patients are often confused about nutrition because they are encouraged to maintain their weight—even if that means eating a high-fat, high-sugar, low-fiber, low-nutrient diet.

While this may be necessary in some cases, current thinking tells us that it's often possible to maintain weight on a diet that emphasizes healthy fats; quality, protein-rich foods; and high-fiber, nutrient-dense foods. These foods also help boost the body's ability to fight disease.

In developing this latest edition of *The Cancer Wellness Cookbook*, we have updated the scientific information on the link between food and cancer and added a variety of delicious and healthy new recipes. Some of the nation's top chefs have shared their favorite recipes with us to include in the book. We've also added recipes from people in the community, cancer patients, cancer survivors, and people working in the cancer field.

♦ **What You Can Expect from** *The Cancer Wellness Cookbook* ♦

* Easy-to-understand descriptions of the key components of good nutrition, including the Top 10 "Super Foods," which may protect and fight against cancer.

* Practical, easy-to-implement suggestions for incorporating healthy eating into your lifestyle.

* A variety of recipes for great-tasting, nutritious dishes that are quick and simple to make, even if you're a novice in the kitchen.

* A helpful resource for caregivers who are trying to make meals that are healthy and appetizing for a cancer patient. Many of these caregivers are spouses who have limited cooking experience.

* Suggestions for reducing the side effects of cancer treatment.

* Help in improving your quality of life and your sense of well-being and control.

* It is important to remember that diet alone is not the sole cause of any cancer, nor is a nutritious diet alone an effective treatment for cancer. It can be a valuable and powerful tool, however, to maintain the highest degree of wellness before, during, and after treatment. Moreover, nutrition and healthy eating may promote survivorship and help prevent cancer recurrence.

* We hope this book assists you in making choices that feel right for you. Happy reading and healthy eating!

ABOUT CANCER LIFELINE

THE WARMTH OF A SMILE ... THE COMFORT OF A HUG ... THE ABSENCE of judgment ... the support of a listening ear ... the healing of laughter ...

That's the essence and the power of Cancer Lifeline. For forty years we have been enriching the lives of those impacted by cancer. We're a nonprofit organization providing cancer patients and their family members, caregivers, friends, and coworkers with the education, resources, and emotional support to live with cancer.

In this spirit of community, Cancer Lifeline was founded in 1973 by a cancer survivor and a group of her close friends who began a twenty-four-hour telephone "Lifeline." We served about 250 people that first year. Since then, our services have grown beyond our wildest dreams: now we serve about twenty thousand people each year.

At our warm, welcoming facility, the Dorothy S. O'Brien Center, our clients can choose classes ranging from exercise, yoga, and meditation to writing, painting, and nutrition. In addition to our programs, we offer individual and family support, resource referrals, and support groups.

In 1996, we published the first edition of this cookbook in an effort to empower cancer patients, caregivers, and others to actively participate in creating nutrition plans with healthy meals. *The Cancer Wellness Cookbook*, our newest edition, contains the latest science about nutrition and cancer, in clear, easy-to-understand language, and offers tasty new recipes focused on the key ingredients that encourage optimal health.

We've designed this book to give you a wealth of information and ideas about nutrition, cooking, and eating. We invite you to choose from it whatever makes sense for nourishing you on your healing journey.

FOR MORE INFORMATION ABOUT CANCER LIFELINE

If you'd like to talk to a caring, trained volunteer on our twenty-four-hour Lifeline, call 206-297-2500 or 1-800-255-5505. Our volunteers offer support, information, and a listening ear. Our Lifeline is a place to seek in-the-moment support for anyone touched by cancer, including patients and their friends, families, or coworkers. Trained staff and volunteers are available to provide warm, nonjudgmental support at your convenience, seven days a week.

We also invite you to visit our website at CancerLifeline.org. Or you may call our business office at 206-297-2100.

Cancer Lifeline: Forty years of providing strength, dignity, and hope to those affected by cancer.

WHAT TO EAT AND DO NOW

FOR PEOPLE WHO ARE LIVING WITH CANCER OR PEOPLE WHO WANT TO protect against cancer, there are clear and helpful guidelines to answer the question "What do I eat now?" In addition to proper nutrition, the scientific community has helped us understand other important lifestyle factors that affect cancer risk and survivorship.

In a landmark study by the American Institute for Cancer Research (AICR) and World Cancer Research Fund (WCRF), an international panel of experts reviewed more than forty-five hundred research studies to determine the relationship between food, nutrition, lifestyle, and cancer. Based on that report and continuous research updates, these experts determined guidelines for what to eat, healthy body weight, and physical activity.

FOLLOW A PLANT-BASED DIET

What is the optimum diet for persons living with cancer? Nutritional guidelines from both the American Cancer Society (ACS) and AICR recommend a plant-based diet.

To understand what a plant-based diet is, picture your plate as two-thirds or more plant-derived foods and one-third or less animal-derived foods. The unique compounds in plant-based foods form their wide range of colors and act as cell-protective nutrients that may derail cancer's progression. Put a medley of colors on your plate to receive the maximum benefits: dark green vegetables like kale and broccoli, red and blue fruits like cherries and blueberries, and yellow-orange vegetables like carrots and winter squash. Try to eat at least five servings of a variety of nonstarchy vegetables and fruits daily.

A plant-based diet is also rich in various whole grains and legumes (beans). Whole grains include brown rice, oats, cracked wheat, kasha, millet, and bulgur. Legumes, like soybeans, black beans, black-eyed peas, and garbanzo beans, are rich sources of fiber and protein.

Processed foods have high amounts of sugar, fat, and salt. These foods are energy-dense (lots of calories in small amounts) but nutrient-poor (lacking fiber and other important compounds). ACS and AICR guidelines recommend limiting sugary drinks and other processed foods.

Eat Select Meats

To supplement the plant foods, small quantities of meats should also be consumed. Choose fish and poultry more often than red meat (beef, lamb, pork). Red meat contains heme iron, nitrite, sodium, and compounds called heterocyclic amines that appear to contribute to cancer risk. Processed meats—like ham, bacon, salami, hot dogs, and sausages—should be avoided. They are clearly linked to colon cancer and may be linked to pancreatic, prostate, and esophageal cancers.

Maintain a Healthy Weight

For cancer survivors and for prevention of cancer and cancer recurrence, both the AICR report and recommendations by the ACS reiterate that achieving and maintaining a healthy weight is a top priority. According to these experts, a healthy weight means that people should be as lean as possible without being underweight. Excess body weight is linked with several types of cancer, including colon and rectal cancer, kidney cancer, and breast cancer in post-menopausal women.

Engage in Physical Activity

To meet the goals of physical activity for cancer survivors, adults should get thirty minutes of activity of any kind each day. Research on survivors of cancers—including breast, colon, prostate, and ovarian cancers—showed that physical activity after diagnosis helped avoid disease recurrence and improved survival rates.

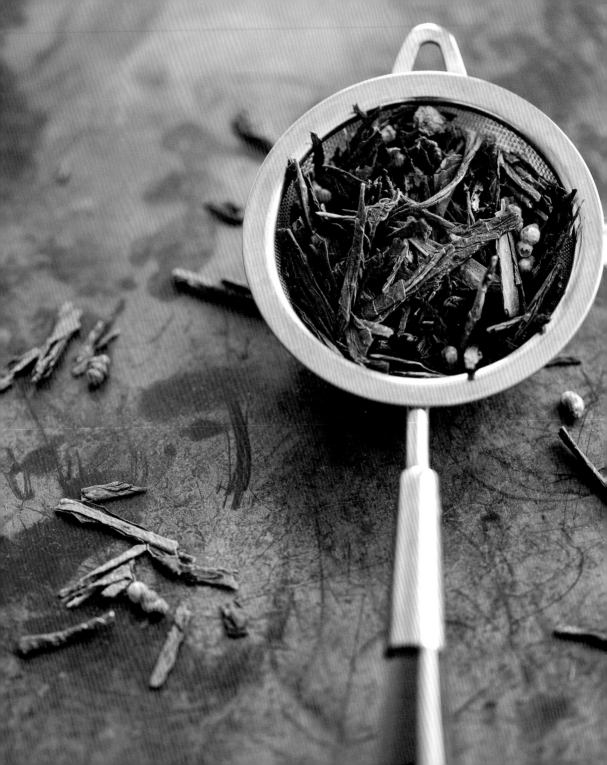

THE TOP 10 "SUPER FOODS"

THE RECOMMENDATION FOR ADOPTING A DIET FOCUSED ON PLANT-based foods stems from the findings that they may help our bodies fight cancer. Plant-based foods help protect cells from damage that causes normal cells to become cancerous. Compounds in these foods—including vitamins, minerals, and phytochemicals—support the body's defenses and help prevent replication of cancerous cells as well as their migration. These same compounds also work to turn on tumor-suppressing genes. Finally, plant-based foods are anti-inflammatory; this is significant because low-level chronic inflammation increases the cascade of cellular changes that may promote cancer.

Phytochemicals (*phyto* is a Greek word that means *plant*) are naturally occurring substances that act as natural defense systems in plants, protecting the plants from infections and from the invasion of disease-causing microorganisms. Phytochemicals (also called phytonutrients) provide plants with an abundance of aromas, colors, and flavors.

Foods rich in phytochemicals show potential for reducing the risk of cancer and cardiovascular disease in humans. Phytochemicals in fruits and vegetables have been shown to reduce cancer risk by regulating detoxification enzymes and stimulating the immune system.

Other phytochemicals in foods help ward off heart disease by making blood platelets "slippery" and thus reducing the chance that these cells will get sticky, clump together, and produce clots that may lead to heart attacks.

Phytochemicals work in a number of ways to prevent or suppress cancer. These compounds in plants boost the activities of the body's enzyme systems that detoxify potential cancer-causing substances (carcinogens), block the action of carcinogens on their target organs or tissue, or act on cells to suppress cancer development.

In addition to being rich sources of phytochemicals, plant-based foods contain other compounds, including antioxidants and fiber, that work to reduce inflammation and bolster the immune system. Inflammation is a key player in the production of compounds that can lead to tumor initiation, growth, and invasion.

Our list of the Top 10 "Super Foods" represents the best choices of phytochemical-rich and anti-inflammatory foods that are proven to help protect against disease and promote good health. All fruits and vegetables are health-building foods, but current research has shown that some are more effective at protecting cells from cancer and inflammation than others. According to nutrition experts, vegetables have more scientific support as cancer preventers than fruits, possibly because they have more cancer-inhibiting phytochemicals.

Adding the Top 10 foods, as well as a variety of other plant-based foods, to your diet is a great step toward better health, whether you're currently in cancer treatment, a cancer survivor, or just a person who's committed to living a healthier life. Throughout this section, you'll find tips for putting the foods to good use, and many of our recipes include these foods as ingredients.

A final note: When buying or growing fruits and vegetables, consider going organic. Organic produce is grown without the use of chemical fertilizers or synthetic insecticides and herbicides; organic meat comes from animals not treated with antibiotics, hormones, or medications. By avoiding foods that come in contact with these harmful chemicals, you reduce your exposure to them as well. A leading researcher on organic foods concluded that data shows pesticide dietary risk is virtually eliminated from organically farmed food. Another bonus? According to 43 percent of people who buy organic foods, they taste better than their conventional counterparts.

Note: If you are currently in treatment, some of the Top 10 "Super Foods" may not sound appealing at the moment. That's okay. Just wait and, when you are ready, add them to your meals and snacks.

1. Broccoli, Cabbage, Cauliflower, and Other Cruciferous Vegetables

POSSIBLE BENEFITS

Vegetables in the cabbage family (called cruciferous vegetables) are rich in cell-protective phytochemicals. These phytochemicals, called glucosinolates, give these vegetables their "bite," act to protect healthy cells from damage, and block the activation of carcinogens.

> **Cruciferous vegetables include:**
> broccoli, cabbage (red, white, napa, and savoy), cauliflower, brussels sprouts, kale, Swiss chard, parsnips, watercress, radishes, bok choy, collard greens, kohlrabi, rutabaga, turnips, and mustard greens.

Foods in this family of vegetables also contain another phytochemical compound called sulphoraphane, which has anti-inflammatory effects and promotes apoptosis (cell death) of cancer cells.

Researchers have found that people who eat more broccoli, cabbage, and cauliflower reduce their risk of colon cancer, and in survivors may block the progression of prostate cancer.

OPTIMIZING CRUCIFEROUS VEGETABLES

Select fresh, organically grown vegetables when they are available. For convenience, keep a supply of frozen broccoli, cauliflower, brussels sprouts, and other cruciferous vegetables on hand.

Broccoli and cauliflower are delicious raw or lightly steamed and can be used with dips or added to salads. Kale, bok choy, and collards are best eaten

THE TOP 10 "SUPER FOODS"

Tomatoes

Fish

Broccoli, cabbage, cauliflower, and other cruciferous vegetables

Nuts and seeds, especially flaxseed

Carotenoid-rich (deep orange, yellow, red, and green) vegetables

Culinary herbs and spices

Green and black teas

Mushrooms

Beans, especially soybeans

Berries and cherries

lightly steamed, added to soups, or used in a medley of vegetables for a colorful stir-fry. Peel and dice kohlrabi—which tastes like a mild, sweet turnip—and eat it as a raw snack, or toss it into a steamed vegetable medley. Try the recipes for Broccoli with Sesame-Crusted Tofu, page 148, or Indian-Style Roasted Cauliflower, page 141.

If you need to have these vitamin-rich vegetables very well cooked during treatment, put them in a soup or puree them in a blender for a creamy, easy-to-digest, and healthful meal.

2. Beans, Especially Soybeans

POSSIBLE BENEFITS

Beans are legumes, the technical term for the family of plants that includes pinto beans, black beans, lentils, and soybeans. Beans are rich in such cancer-fighting phytochemicals as saponins, protease inhibitors, and phytic acid.

Saponins are compounds in beans that help keep normal cells from turning into cancer cells and that prevent cancer cells from growing. Other compounds in beans, such as protease inhibitors, protect plants against attacks by viruses and other disease-causing agents.

Cancer researchers have determined that protease inhibitors are extremely potent agents with the ability to suppress the cancer process. Phytic acid, another beneficial compound in beans, may help to enhance immunity and works as an antioxidant to neutralize cell-damaging free radicals.

Beans of all varieties are an outstanding source of fiber. The fiber from beans nourish and support friendly bacteria in the gut that stimulate the immune system. Fiber-rich diets may also prevent unfriendly, disease-causing bacteria from flourishing. Fiber from beans helps prevent constipation—one of the possible side effects of cancer treatment. They are also excellent sources of protein, calcium, potassium, zinc, and iron.

Soybeans and Other Soy Foods

The ancient Chinese considered soy, which is native to eastern Asia, to be one of the five sacred grains vital for life. Soy protein is nutritionally equivalent to proteins derived from animal sources, including eggs, milk, and meat. Soy foods include tofu, tempeh, miso, soy milk, edamame beans, and whole soybeans.

Soy foods contain phytoestrogens (very weak versions of human estrogen) that act as antioxidants, carcinogen blockers, or tumor suppressors. Isoflavones are one class of these phytoestrogens in soy foods. These substances regulate hormone function in both women and men and may exert a protective effect against hormone-related tumors such as breast and prostate cancer.

Asian populations are known to have a low incidence of breast, prostate, and other cancers. Epidemiologists hypothesize that this may be attributable to the average daily intake of one serving of soy (equal to approximately 40 milligrams of isoflavones).

If you're a breast cancer survivor, you may wonder whether you can safely eat soy foods. Human studies show that isoflavones in soy do not increase risk of recurrence for breast cancer. With this evidence, leading researchers have concluded that it is safe to eat soy in moderate amounts—up to three servings per day.

Optimizing Beans

Beans make wonderful, inexpensive additions to soups, salads, stews, pastas, and casseroles. Easy, flavorful dips and spreads can be made with garbanzo, black, or pinto beans (try the Lickety-Split Hummus, page 118). For a healthy and fast meal, heat a can of beans with some tomato sauce and seasonings. Have fun experimenting with various herbs and spices mixed into different kinds of beans. Be adventurous!

One serving of soy equals:

* 1 cup soy milk
* ½ cup tofu
* ½ cup whole soybeans
* ½ cup green soybeans (edamame), edible parts
* ¼ cup soy nuts
* ½ cup tempeh
* 2 tablespoons miso

If you're just getting friendly with soy foods, try soy milk on your cereal. Soy milk and other soy products are readily available in your grocery store or natural foods supermarket. Another great idea is to add tofu to the Yogurt Protein Shake, page 86.

Edamame beans make a quick, fiber- and protein-rich snack ready in just a few minutes. Look for edamame—also called green soybeans—in bags in the freezer section of the supermarket; you can buy them shelled or in their pods. Marinated or seasoned packaged tofu makes a great addition to stir-fry dishes, or you can slice it and stuff it inside pita bread for a quick grab-and-go meal. Swapping beef for a soy burger or cooking soy sausage or breakfast patties with brunch are other easy ways to incorporate soy into your meals.

Add beans to your diet gradually so your digestive tract has a chance to adjust. The average person can start out by eating half a cup of beans every two or three days, gradually working up to a cup or more per day. In recipes calling for beans, try substituting soybeans for half of the total beans.

3. Berries and Cherries

POSSIBLE BENEFITS

A variety of berries and cherries contain powerful antioxidant compounds called anthocyanins that protect cells from damage by free radicals. Damaged cells that are not neutralized by antioxidants can replicate and begin the cancer process. Anthocyanins in berries may also affect how genes and molecular pathways are triggered in our bodies. These compounds can help these pathways express delay signals rather than promotion signals for cancer development. The blue, blue-red, and purple colors in fruits such as blueberries, cherries, grapes, raspberries, and cranberries are produced by anthocyanins. In addition to anthocyanins, berries contain elegiac acid, another anticancer compound.

OPTIMIZING BERRIES

Toss fresh or frozen berries into a smoothie, add them to your breakfast cereal, mix some into a fruit salad, or just snack on them. Mix and match your berries for maximum benefit. Fresh, seasonal berries are usually available from May through September. The rest of the year, buy frozen berries. Try our recipe for Simply Delicious Berries, page 222, or Blueberry Breakfast Cake, page 95, for tasty ways to eat your anthocyanins.

4. Culinary Herbs and Spices

POSSIBLE BENEFITS

Herbs and spices are not only prized for adding a wide range of flavors and colors to foods, but are valued for their potential health benefits. Rich in antioxidants, these foods may help cancer cell death and suppress potential carcinogens. One researcher identified more than 180 compounds in spices that may provide health benefits. Scientists have explored the anticancer action of herbs and spices including basil, caraway, cardamom, cinnamon, clove, coriander, cumin, garlic, ginger, rosemary, saffron, thyme, and turmeric. Turmeric, ginger, and garlic (which is part of the onion family) have both anti-inflammatory and antioxidant benefits.

Turmeric contains curcumin, the subject of extensive research for its effect on a number of cancers. Curcumin ranks high in an index of anti-inflammatory foods. In studies of people with a genetic disease that causes the growth of hundreds of polyps (pre-cancerous growths) in the colon, curcumin dramatically decreased both the number and size of the polyps.

Ginger, an herb in the same family as turmeric, also has a high ranking among anti-inflammatory foods. In animal studies, ginger acts as both an antioxidant and anti-inflammatory compound by increasing liver enzymes that defuse potential carcinogens. Ginger may also be helpful as an antinausea compound. In one study, patients were given standard antinausea medication with either ginger or a placebo. Ginger was taken twice daily for six days, starting three days prior to chemotherapy. Researchers reported that compared to patients who took the placebo with medication, patients taking ginger with medication experienced significantly reduced nausea.

Garlic is an allium in the onion family. Garlic is rich in sulfur, which is the backbone of antioxidant compounds formed in the body to protect healthy cells. Human studies on the action of garlic on cancer show a reduction in the development of stomach cancer in high-risk people. Animal studies show "compelling" evidence that garlic may lower incidence of breast, colon, skin, and lung cancers.

Optimizing Culinary Herbs and Spices

Be bold with herbs. Try adding turmeric to vegetables, such as in the Curried Root Vegetables, page 139. Experiment with curries (turmeric-rich spice combinations) in a recipe like Spicy Chickpea, Kale, and Tomato Stew, page 200. Make Ginger Tea, page 49, to help with chemotherapy-related nausea. You can also combine two powerhouse superfoods, garlic and ginger, in a marinade such as the one featured in Broccoli with Sesame-Crusted Tofu, page 148. Or keep it simple and try roasting garlic bulbs to eat as an appetizer spread on whole grain crackers or to serve as a vegetable side with dinner.

5. Carotenoid-Rich (Deep Orange, Yellow, Red, and Green) Produce

POSSIBLE BENEFITS

While all produce is good for you, a number of fruits and vegetables contain compounds called carotenoids that may protect against rapid cell production, which can increase the risk of cancer. The way that carotenoids protect healthy cells and fortify the immune system may be related to formation of another form of vitamin A, called retinol. Foods high in carotenoids protect against cancers of the mouth, pharynx, larynx, and lung.

Eat any of the carotenoid-rich foods as often as you like. Many fresh fruits and vegetables can be washed, cut up, and stored in airtight containers so you'll have plenty of healthy raw produce readily accessible for snacking on or cooking.

Carotenoids are present in deep orange, green, yellow, and red vegetables and fruits. They contain antioxidants, compounds that are important in fighting free radicals—the by-products of the natural activity of oxygen in cells. Free radicals are very reactive and roam the body, damaging cells and the genetic material within them. This can hinder the natural ability of cells to resist the development of cancer.

Our cells have well-developed systems for fighting free radicals and mending the damage they cause, and we can assist the cells by eating an antioxidant-rich, plant-based diet. Many studies have reported a relationship between low risk for cancer and high consumption of foods containing antioxidants.

OPTIMIZING CAROTENOID-RICH PRODUCE

Add a rainbow of brightly colored fruits and vegetables to your meals and snacks. In the vegetable family, yams, winter squash, and sweet potatoes deliver the highest amount of carotenoids actually absorbed by the body.

Other sources of carotenoid include bok choy, broccoli, carrots, corn, greens (collards, kale, lettuce, spinach), pumpkin, bell peppers, tomatoes, and tomato products. Fruits such as apricots, cantaloupe, nectarines, peaches, oranges, papayas, and watermelon are also excellent sources of carotenoids. Gingered Carrot Soup, page 136, and Baked Sweet Potato Fries, page 143, deliver these nutrients with wonderful flavor.

6. Fish

POSSIBLE BENEFITS

Fish is rich in omega-3 fatty acids—healthy fats that may have a role in the prevention of colon cancer. Researchers studied cancer risk in men based on how frequently they ate fish, including tuna, salmon, sardines, and others. The men who ate fish five times or more per week had a 40 percent lower risk of developing colon cancer than those who ate fish less than once per week.

Fish seems to protect against cancer by restricting the production of prostaglandins—inflammatory compounds that act as tumor promoters. Research scientists found that DHA (one of the compounds in fish) reduced solid tumor size and boosted the effect of the chemotherapy drug cisplatin.

Eating fish is also good for your heart. The American Heart Association recommends that adults eat at least two servings of fish per week. The fish that are highest in omega-3 fatty acids include mackerel, salmon, sardines, rainbow trout, herring, and albacore tuna. Cod, flounder, clams, catfish, haddock, perch, and halibut have lower amounts of omega-3s.

OPTIMIZING FISH

Make a habit of eating fish frequently, poached, baked, or lightly sautéed with some garlic. Go for convenience if your energy resources are limited: purchase foil-packed or canned fish and use it in salads, add it to a sandwich, or just eat it plain as a snack. Add the Salmon with Sun-Dried Tomato Sauce, page 175, or Pan-Seared Petrale Sole with Lemon-Caper-Butter Sauce, page 171, to your menus for delicious ways to eat more fish.

7. Tomatoes

POSSIBLE BENEFITS

Tomatoes contain lycopene, a phytochemical that has several anticancer effects. Lycopene acts as a potent antioxidant to stop free radicals from tearing through the body's cell membranes and harming the DNA. This phytonutrient also helps to restore the normal cellular communication that is lacking in tumors. When the cells are able to communicate, cancer cells can be signaled to halt their growth.

In Mediterranean countries, where people eat a lot of tomatoes as well as other fruits and vegetables, there are lower cancer rates. One study showed that when men ate ten or more servings of tomato products per week, they experienced a 35 percent reduction in prostate cancer. The effects were even stronger with more advanced or aggressive prostate cancer. Lycopene also appears to be effective against breast cancer.

Processed tomato products such as spaghetti sauce and tomato paste, puree, and juice have two to eight times more lycopene than raw tomatoes. Other produce that contains lycopene includes watermelon, pink grapefruit, apricots, and pink guavas.

OPTIMIZING TOMATOES AND OTHER LYCOPENE-RICH FOODS

Enjoy a rich tomato sauce on your steamed vegetables. Drink tomato juice as a snack. Make a nourishing dish like Basil-Spiked Tomato Soup, page 122, and add a quick and easy mini pizza on the side: top an English muffin with tomato sauce, lightly steamed veggies, and a sprinkle of low-fat cheese. Snack on grapefruit, apricots, or watermelon slices.

8. Mushrooms

POSSIBLE BENEFITS

Mushrooms have been revered in Asia as potent medicines for thousands of years. In fact, Chinese emperors and Japanese royalty drank mushroom teas and concoctions to achieve vitality and long life. Mushrooms are low in calories and carbohydrates and rich in vegetable proteins and essential amino acids. They are a source of some fiber and contain a number of important vitamins and minerals, including B vitamins, iron, potassium, selenium, and zinc.

White button mushrooms, readily available and less costly than other varieties of mushrooms, show potent anticancer properties. Using extracts from the mushrooms, researchers found that button mushrooms inhibited aromatase activity in breast cancer cell lines. White button mushrooms showed better aromatase-blocking action than shiitake, portobello, and cremini mushrooms. Other mushrooms, including shiitake and maitake, contain polysaccharides—substances that may stimulate the immune system and provide anticancer protection. Polysaccharides may increase the production of immune system defenders such as cytokines and macrophages, which recognize and destroy cancer cells, viruses, and bacteria.

Shiitake mushrooms contain a form of polysaccharide called lentinan, a substance that appears to stimulate the body's own antioxidant defense system and activate the immune system. Animals given lentinan derived from shiitake mushrooms developed significantly smaller tumors than those not receiving it.

The maitake mushroom, also known as hen-of-the-woods or dancing mushroom, contains a polysaccharide compound called beta-glucan or D-fraction. Beta-glucan appears to increase the action of natural killer (NK) cells, which regulate immune system responses and cause the death of tumor cells.

Studies on the protective qualities of shiitake, maitake, and other mushrooms have used only compounds extracted from mushrooms, so it's unknown whether eating fresh mushrooms in relatively small quantities will provide any protective effects. Nevertheless, mushrooms are a healthy, nutritious food that may have medicinal properties, so enjoy the many delicious and intriguing varieties.

OPTIMIZING MUSHROOMS

Mushrooms have a wonderful, meaty texture and can be added to stir-fries, soups, or casseroles. Arame-Stuffed Mushroom Caps, page 144, make an elegant addition to any meal or party. Try different mushrooms in soups, like Shiitake Mushroom and Lentil Soup, page 128, or Black Bean Soup, page 132, which includes white button mushrooms. Most large grocery stores carry several mushroom varieties, including shiitake and maitake.

---

9. Nuts and Seeds, Especially Flaxseed

POSSIBLE BENEFITS

Nuts are nutritional wonders. They provide concentrated energy in small "packages" that contain protein, fats, and fiber. Brazil nuts, almonds, cashews, and walnuts contain about 6 grams of protein in ⅓ cup, as well as 1 to 2 grams of fiber. Nuts are excellent sources of cancer-fighting and anti-inflammatory vitamins and minerals including magnesium, selenium, and vitamin E.

Nuts and nut butters are excellent choices during cancer treatments, when eating may be a challenge. A small amount of nuts goes a long way, though: just ⅓ cup has 240 to 300 calories. Nuts are high in fat, but it's mostly the healthier form: unsaturated fat.

Nuts appear to have a positive effect on prostate cancer. Researchers who studied data on men from fifty-nine countries found that as consumption of nuts and seeds increased, mortality from prostate cancer decreased.

Walnuts contain omega-3 fatty acids, carotenoids, and vitamin E. One or all of these compounds may slow cancer growth. In animal studies, walnuts slowed the growth of colon cancer by halting the formation of blood lines that feed tumors (a process called angiogenesis). In another study, mice who were engineered to develop prostate cancer and fed walnut-rich diets (about 2.8 ounces of walnuts per day) had a 28 percent lower rate of tumor growth. Walnuts have also been shown to lower LDL (bad) cholesterol.

Flax and flaxseed contain several important health-protective substances, including fiber (more fiber than in oat bran) and alpha-linolenic acid, an omega-3 fatty acid that is linked to a lower risk of heart disease and cancer.

Flaxseed is a rich source of lignans, compounds that are transformed by the bacteria in our bodies into compounds that may protect against tumor formation and growth. Lignans in flaxseed protected mice exposed to radiation, and the animals with the highest intake of lignans had the least weight loss and a longer survival time. Researchers have also found that flaxseed reduces tumor size and numbers in animals and humans. Estrogen-receptor-negative breast cancer patients who ate a daily muffin containing 25 grams of flaxseed for thirty-nine days experienced reduced breast tumor growth.

Tip from Jeanne, a cancer survivor:
"I put ground flaxseed on everything. I make muffins with added flaxseed and eat one every day."

In addition, flaxseed (30 grams a day) and a low-fat diet (20 percent fat) lowered prostate-specific antigen (PSA) levels in prostate cancer patients after an average treatment time of thirty-four days.

OPTIMIZING NUTS AND FLAXSEED

Sprinkle chopped nuts on cereal, stir them into yogurt, or add some to your favorite salad. Toss nuts into stir-fries and pastas. Experiment with different types of nuts in a beloved muffin or pancake recipe. Spread almond, peanut, or other nut butters on bread and waffles.

Flaxseed can be purchased as whole seeds, meal, flour, or oil. You can grind the seeds into a meal at home using a coffee mill or spice grinder. Sprinkle ground flaxseed on cereal or salads, or mix it into soups. Flaxseed can also be added to muffins, breads, and cookies.

10. Green and Black Teas

POSSIBLE BENEFITS

Both green and black teas, but not herbal teas, contain phytochemicals called polyphenols and related compounds. These compounds act as powerful antioxidants and may also limit cell replication, a primary characteristic of cancer.

Polyphenols in tea are known to inhibit compounds that are involved in tumor survival and metastasis. They also thwart the activities of many tumor-associated compounds that drive cell growth.

♦ Best Use of Flaxseed for Women Taking Tamoxifen or Aromatase Inhibitors ♦

In animal studies, flaxseed did not interfere with tamoxifen's actions and may actually increase the effectiveness of tamoxifen. However, to date, there have been no clinical trials on flaxseed and tamoxifen or aromatase inhibitors. To make the best decision about whether or not to add flaxseed to your diet, keep updated on the latest research. Check websites such as the American Institute for Cancer Research (aicr.org) and consult with your health care provider. If you decide to eat flaxseed, do so in moderation—about 1 tablespoon or 10 grams a day.

If you have prostate cancer, ground flaxseed is a better choice than flaxseed oil. Flaxseed contains lignans that appear to bind to testosterone and decrease circulating levels of this hormone, which is a good thing for prostate cancer. Consume about 2 tablespoons of the ground seed daily.

Compounds in green tea, such as polyphenols, help eliminate free radicals that can alter DNA, causing cell mutation and leading to cancer formation. Researchers who reviewed population studies found that increased green tea intake may reduce risk of breast cancer recurrence.

Inflammation is positively associated with many forms of cancer, including prostate. Men with prostate cancer who drank six cups of green tea daily three to eight weeks before scheduled prostate surgery had reduced markers of inflammation and significantly lower PSA levels.

OPTIMIZING GREEN AND BLACK TEAS

Make tea your beverage of choice. Enjoy a cup with your breakfast, and make your caffeine count: green tea has health benefits with only moderate amounts of caffeine, and even decaffeinated green tea provides the benefits of the phytochemicals. Start your own teatime—take a late-afternoon break with a cup of tea. In the summer, brew iced green tea for a refreshing pick-me-up. Black tea is also a good option, though it doesn't have the same strength of anticancer compounds like catechins as green tea. A word of warning: Don't drink tea that is too hot; it may increase the risk of esophageal cancer. Green tea may interact with medications that you are taking, so discuss this with your health care advisor.

NUTRIENTS THAT PROMOTE GOOD HEALTH

GETTING ALL THE NUTRIENTS YOUR BODY NEEDS TO RUN OPTIMALLY is important for everyone, but it's especially important for cancer survivors. As your body is recovering from disease, it needs all the help it can get to repair and rebuild healthy tissue. Because eating may be more difficult during recovery, it is advantageous to pack as many nutrients as possible into the foods you do consume.

Your body requires six basic nutrients. Water is the nutrient needed in the greatest quantity, followed by protein, carbohydrates, fat, vitamins, and minerals. Protein, carbohydrates, and fat are called macronutrients because your body needs them in large quantities. Vitamins and minerals are called micronutrients because they are needed in smaller amounts.

WATER

You may not think of water as one of the key nutrients, but it is. Water makes up approximately 50 to 60 percent of the body's weight. It brings to your body's cells the exact nutrients they need and carries away waste products.

Water helps your body digest food, transport other nutrients, maintain normal body temperature, flush toxins, and remove waste products. Fatigue, a common side effect of cancer treatment, can be exacerbated by not drinking enough fluids. Your body excretes approximately 3 quarts of water every day. To replace that water, drink at least 2 quarts of fluids throughout the day. (You may need more fluids if you're on chemotherapy, or less if your sodium

27

level is out of balance. Your nurse, doctor, or registered dietitian can advise you on the amount that's right for you.) You can consume another quart of water simply by eating plenty of fruits and vegetables.

To meet your fluids quota, choose water, mineral waters (without added sodium), bottled water flavored with fruit essence (without added sugars), or fruit juice diluted with sparkling water. Caffeine-free herbal tea is also a good choice. Many people like to keep a bottle of water with them at all times to make drinking more convenient.

Limit your consumption of sodas (especially caffeinated ones), coffee, and alcohol. They may have a dehydrating effect that can rob your body of fluids.

> **Tip from Jeanne, a cancer survivor:** "When I was on chemo, I added flavorings like lemon or mint to water to hide the metallic taste."

MACRONUTRIENTS

The macronutrients—protein, fat, and carbohydrates—are the body's primary sources of fuel, and they also play a major role in maintaining the balance of many of the hormones and enzymes in the body. Two of those hormones, insulin and glucagon, control the sugar levels in the blood and the enzymes that balance the body's metabolic processes. These metabolic processes produce energy, help regulate your immune system, and control many other body functions.

A diet that provides a healthy balance of macronutrients is especially important if your body has been stressed or compromised by disease and its treatment.

Protein: The Body's Building Blocks

The body uses protein to build, maintain, and repair tissue. It helps regulate many of the body's chemical processes. Normal protein intake is about 56 grams a day for men, 46 grams for women. However, during cancer treatment your body is under a great deal of stress, so you may need more protein—80 grams or more each day—to repair and rebuild tissue and help prevent infection.

How much protein do you need? Protein needs vary from person to person, and your need will probably fluctuate as you progress through treatment and recovery. Work with a registered dietician or your nurse or doctor to determine your optimal protein intake before, during, and after treatment.

Sources of Protein

Most of the foods we eat contain some protein, but some foods have more protein than others. Here are a few examples.

> ◆ **Caution: Red Meat** ◆
>
> Eating large quantities of red meat is positively associated with colon cancer, heart disease, stroke, and diabetes. So how much red meat is safe to eat? The American Institute for Cancer Research recommends eating no more than 18 ounces (cooked weight) per week of red meats like beef, lamb, and pork. These guidelines also suggest avoiding processed meats such as ham, bacon, salami, hot dogs, and sausages.

ABOUT 7 GRAMS OF PROTEIN:
1 ounce lean meat, poultry, or fish
½ cup legumes
¼ cup tofu
1 cup broccoli or brussels sprouts
½ cup cottage cheese
1 cup egg noodles
7 ounces milk or yogurt
1 ounce cheese
2 tablespoons peanut butter

1 large egg
1 to 2 ounces nuts or seeds

ABOUT 3 GRAMS OF PROTEIN:
⅓ cup cooked rice
½ cup cooked cereal or grains
1 slice bread

ABOUT 2 GRAMS OF PROTEIN:
1 cup raw vegetables
½ cup cooked vegetables

As you choose protein sources, remember that the goal is to choose moderate portions of animal protein and experiment with consuming more plant-based proteins such as legumes. Good choices for animal proteins include skinless chicken and turkey, fish and shellfish, lean cuts of red meat (round, loin, or flank), eggs, low-fat and nonfat cheeses, and other low-fat and nonfat dairy products such as yogurt and milk.

Plant proteins—which include beans, nuts and seeds, and some grains—provide quality protein and add variety to your meals. Make liberal use of legumes, grains, and vegetables in your diet. Other excellent sources of plant protein include tofu and other soy products, dried beans, brown rice, barley, and nuts such as almonds and walnuts.

Legumes are the fruit or seeds of leguminous plants. They include kidney beans, soybeans, split peas, lentils, black-eyed peas, and lima beans. Their specially adapted root systems trap nitrogen in the soil and turn it into compounds that become part of the seed. The result? Legumes are richer in high-quality protein than most plant foods.

The notion that plant foods need to be specially combined at each meal to make "complete" protein is outdated. The body pools and stores amino acids from foods in muscle and other tissues and uses them to assemble proteins as needed.

Experiment with creating meals that emphasize plant proteins. Some winning combinations include:

- Beans, salsa, and low-fat cheese wrapped in a tortilla
- Bread and peanut butter with your favorite add-in (such as a sliced banana)
- Tofu and vegetable stir-fry
- Bean and vegetable soup combined with green salad or crusty bread

Carbohydrates: The Body's Preferred Fuel

CARBOHYDRATES are the body's primary source of immediate fuel. They offer a wide variety of nutrients that nourish the brain and central nervous system, provide energy, and help keep bowel movements regular. Fiber found in whole foods such as fruits, vegetables, beans, and grains stimulates the muscles of the digestive tract so that they retain their health and tone. This in turn speeds up the transit time of materials—including those linked with cancer—through the colon. Fiber also maintains bowel health and may reduce the incidence of colon cancer.

OPTIMAL CARBOHYDRATES are whole foods and minimally processed foods that contain all their fiber and vitamins. They have many components, so it takes time for them to be broken down and reach your bloodstream. They make the best all-around fuel because they "burn" slowly and can help increase your feelings of stamina.

HIGHLY PROCESSED CARBOHYDRATES, on the other hand, have had their fiber and vitamins removed and are digested and absorbed into the bloodstream more quickly. They don't provide the feelings of stamina and endurance that complex carbohydrates do. In fact, they promote greater increases in blood sugar and insulin levels, which can lead to increased fatigue.

Sources of Carbohydrates

The best sources of optimal carbohydrates are dried beans and peas; unprocessed grains such as brown rice, polenta, and quinoa; whole grain breads, cereals, and pastas; and fruits and vegetables.

Limit your intake of highly processed carbohydrates such as baked goods that contain a lot of sugar, sweetened cereals made from white flour rather than whole grains, candy, and soda. Try to use less white rice and pasta made from white flours.

> During treatment, some foods, including beans or nuts and seeds, may be harder to digest. You can add these foods back into your diet after your treatment.

Fat: Making the Best Choices

The body is constantly using small amounts of fat for fuel. Fat in moderate amounts is essential for good health. Although all types of fat have similar amounts of calories, eating healthier fats—particularly plant-based fats and omega-3 fatty acids—may promote health benefits such as reduced inflammation and improved blood cholesterol levels.

Types of Fat

UNSATURATED FATS are primarily found in plant foods. Unsaturated fats have beneficial effects on the body because these fats lower inflammation and appear to promote healthy cholesterol levels. Monounsaturated fat comes from plant sources and includes olive, canola, peanut, sesame, avocado, and walnut oils. Nuts and seeds, such as walnuts and pumpkin seeds, fall into this category. Monounsaturated fat, which is liquid at room temperature, reduces only the damaging LDL cholesterol and leaves HDL cholesterol untouched. (LDL cholesterol promotes heart disease but HDL cholesterol protects against heart attacks.)

POLYUNSATURATED FAT comes from plant sources such as corn, soy, and safflower oils and is liquid at room temperature. These fats occur in foods as either omega-3 or omega-6 fatty acids. Researchers found that the men with nonmetastatic prostate cancer who ate more vegetable fats from nuts and oil-based salad dressings had a 26 percent lower risk of death from any cause, including prostate cancer, heart disease, or other cancers. Since most people eat more omega-6 fats than omega-3 fats, using more monounsaturated fats like canola oil, olive oil, or nuts and seeds in your meals can help bring you back to a good balance of omega-6s to omega-3s.

OMEGA-3 FATTY ACIDS are highly polyunsaturated fats found in fish such as salmon and mackerel as well as in leafy vegetables and flaxseed products. These fatty acids have an anticlotting action that may be effective in preventing heart attack and stroke. They may also improve immune function and, in animal studies, have been shown to inhibit tumor growth. The recommended intake of omega-3 fatty acids can be met by eating omega-3-rich fish twice or more per week; these include salmon, sardines, halibut, herring, mackerel, and anchovies. Most other fish—including cod, flounder, tuna, clams, catfish, haddock, perch, and halibut—have smaller amounts of omega-3s.

SATURATED FATS are found in animal sources such as butter, meat, lard, and whole milk products in addition to tropical oils like coconut and palm oils. This type of fat is usually solid at room temperatures. When you focus on nutrient-rich foods like whole grains, fruits and vegetables, nuts, fish, and beans, small amounts of saturated fats can be allowed as part of your eating plan. But when they're consumed in popular processed foods like pizza, cookies, donuts, and cakes, these fats represent empty calories with little nutritional value. Try to limit these foods.

HYDROGENATED FATS (also called trans fats) are polyunsaturated fats that have been chemically changed. In the transformation process, hydrogenated fats lose their unsaturated characters and the health benefits that go with them. Hydrogenated and partially hydrogenated oils are found in commercially prepared baked goods, shortenings, and deep-fried foods. Hydrogenated fats should be avoided as they have inflammatory effects and increase risk factors for heart disease.

Are Your Omega Fats in Balance?

The goal is to consume a diet that provides a balance of omega-6 and omega-3 fatty acids. In the typical American diet, the ratio of omega-6s to omega-3s is estimated to be 10:1. Omega-3 fatty acids have been shown to be anti-inflammatory and may reduce the risk of cancer. Eat at least one serving twice per week of omega-3-rich fatty fish like anchovies, salmon, or halibut. Plant sources of omega-3s should be eaten daily and include canola oil, walnuts, flaxseed, and green vegetables like kale, broccoli, and salad greens.

Desirable Sources of Fat

If you're losing weight and are being encouraged to eat more calories in the form of fat, be sure to select fat that has nutrients. Some ideas: Make a high-calorie shake with reduced-fat milk, soy milk, Greek yogurt, or tofu (see our Yogurt Protein Shake, page 86). Spread peanut butter or other nut butters on bread or waffles. Or add avocado to a sandwich or salad.

Fats are beneficial and play an important role in good nutrition. But fats have more than twice as many calories (9 calories per gram) than protein or carbohydrate (4 calories per gram). If you are overweight, or trying to maintain a healthy weight, practice portion control when eating fats so you don't overdo it. To manage calories, begin choosing low-fat or nonfat milk products; lean broiled, baked, or braised meats; skinless fish and poultry; and fresh fruits and vegetables prepared with small amounts of oil or cream. Try getting more of your protein from plant sources such as dried peas and beans, grains, and vegetables and soy-based products like tofu.

MICRONUTRIENTS

While your body needs micronutrients in smaller quantities than it does macronutrients, each of them is essential to achieving and maintaining good health.

Vitamins: Necessary for Life and Growth

Vitamins are chemical compounds that the body requires in small amounts. While they don't provide energy, they help the body process and use the energy it gets from food. Most vitamins cannot be made by the body or are not made in sufficient quantities to meet the body's needs, so they must be supplied by food.

Diets rich in foods containing antioxidant vitamins—E, C, and beta-carotene (a plant form of vitamin A)—may protect against many forms of cancer, including oral, esophageal, and reproductive-system cancers. Many studies have linked consumption of foods rich in vitamin C with a reduced risk of cancer.

Sources of Vitamins E, C, and Beta-Carotene

Fruits (whole and juices): Citrus, apricots, kiwis, mangoes, peaches, strawberries, cantaloupe and other melons, and papayas
Vegetables (whole and juices): Carrots, broccoli, brussels sprouts, sweet potatoes, red and green peppers, tomatoes, peas, and spinach

Minerals: The Body's Regulators

Minerals are found in all body tissues and fluids. They help the body build tissue, regulate body processes, maintain fluid balance, and use the energy from food. They do not provide energy.

It is essential that we consume enough minerals to ensure the proper functioning of our bodies. For cancer survivors, who may be eating less, it can be difficult to get sufficient quantities of minerals, including potassium, magnesium, zinc, and calcium.

Several studies have suggested that foods high in calcium might help reduce the risk of colorectal cancer, and minerals like selenium have anti-cancer effects that help keep healthy cells from becoming DNA damaged. Researchers found that men who had higher levels of selenium had lower risk of prostate cancer, especially more aggressive prostate cancer.

Treatment and its side effects can result in deficiencies in essential minerals, so try to pack your diet with whole foods—fruits, vegetables, beans, and grains—that can help your body replace them.

Sources of Minerals

The sources of the following minerals are listed from highest to lowest levels of each.

CALCIUM: Collard greens (1 cup, cooked), calcium-fortified orange juice (1 cup), sardines (3 ounces, canned), soy milk (1 cup), cow's milk (1 cup), sea vegetables (dulse: 3 ounces, dried), figs (10 medium), almonds (¼ cup), tofu (½ cup), navy beans (1 cup, cooked), broccoli (1 cup, cooked).

IRON: Tofu (½ cup, firm), baked beans (1 cup), blackstrap molasses (1 table-spoon), spaghetti with tomato sauce (1 cup), apricots (10 halves, dried), spinach (1 cup, fresh), green peas (½ cup, cooked), whole wheat bread (1 slice), roasted chicken breast (1 breast, 3 oz), broccoli (½ cup, cooked).

MAGNESIUM: Kidney beans (½ cup, cooked), spinach (½ cup, cooked), almonds (1 ounce/24 nuts), soybeans (½ cup, cooked), pumpkin seeds (1 ounce/88 seeds), potato (1 medium, cooked), beet greens (½ cup, cooked), broccoli (½ cup, cooked), raspberries (1 cup), carrots (½ cup, cooked).

POTASSIUM: Dates (6, dried), cantaloupe (½ melon), potato (1 medium, cooked), lima beans (½ cup, cooked), banana (1 medium), spinach (½ cup, cooked), broccoli (1 cup, cooked), salmon (4 ounces, canned), tomato (1 medium), peanuts (1 ounce/28 whole peanuts).

SELENIUM: Brazil nuts (1 ounce/6 to 8 whole nuts), fish (including snapper, halibut, salmon, scallops; 3 ounces, baked), sunflower seeds (1 ounce, ¼ cup), whole wheat bread (1 slice).

Sea Vegetables: A Great Source of Minerals

Sea vegetables contain ten to twenty times the minerals of land plants. Sea vegetables such as nori, kombu, hijiki, dulse, and wakame are excellent sources of calcium, magnesium, and potassium—and they add minerals while enriching the flavor of foods. Nori, for example, is one of the richest sea vegetable sources of protein and also contains large amounts of vitamins C, B1, and A.

Adding sea vegetables to your favorite recipes is easy. For dishes that cook longer than an hour, toss in whole or cut-up sea vegetables like kombu or wakame at the beginning of the cooking time. They lend a wonderfully

♦ Boost Iron ♦

To enhance the absorption of iron, add vitamin C–rich foods—kiwi, broccoli, red bell pepper, papaya, and citrus fruits—to your diet.

rich flavor, especially to stews. For dishes that cook for less than an hour, soak the quicker-cooking sea vegetables—like arame—for ten minutes, until soft enough to cut. Then chop and add to the dish. (Try our recipe for Arame-Stuffed Mushroom Caps on page 144.) When eating out, vegetarian nori rolls are a great way to enjoy sea vegetables.

SUPPLEMENTS TO YOUR DIET

It's important to get as many of your daily nutrients as possible from vitamin-rich whole foods, such as fruits, vegetables, beans, and grains. This is because some substances contained in whole foods are not available in supplement form. In fact, there may be important substances in food of which we aren't even aware yet.

Since optimal nutrition is essential when you're fighting disease, taking supplements may be a beneficial choice, especially if you are having difficulty eating. It is believed that good nutrition decreases recovery time, speeds return of the senses of smell and taste to normal, promotes healing of wounds, and helps restore a sense of well-being more quickly.

Talk to your doctor, nurse, or registered dietitian before taking supplements if you're in treatment. High doses of supplements may interfere with chemo or radiation therapy.

◆ Nutrition Tip ◆

Sea vegetables such as nori, kombu, hijiki, and wakame are excellent sources of calcium, magnesium, and potassium. They add minerals while enriching the flavor of foods. Information about ordering sea vegetables is available from Eden Foods (EdenFoods.com) or Ocean Harvest Sea Vegetables (OHSV.net).

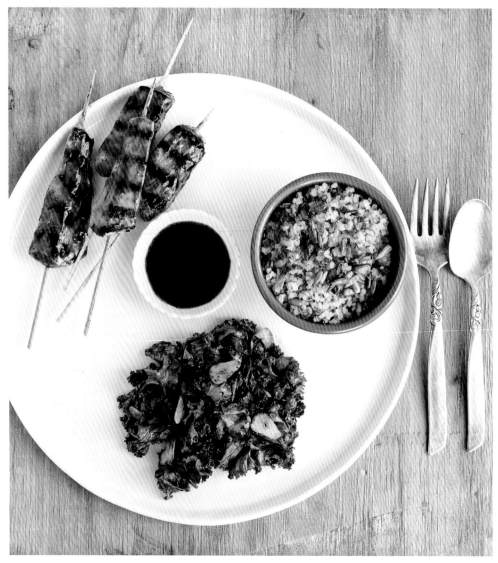

A balanced plate: two-thirds plant foods and one-third or less lean meat, poultry, fish, or low-fat dairy products

CREATING A HEALTHIER DIET

WE HAVE DISCUSSED THE BENEFITS OF EATING A PRIMARILY PLANT-based diet featuring fruits, vegetables, beans, nuts and seeds, and whole grains, and including the Top 10 "Super Foods." We've also covered the basic building blocks of nutrition, including fats, carbohydrates, proteins, vitamins, and minerals.

How do we put all these components together to create a healthier diet? Picture your plate with two-thirds plant foods and one-third or less lean meat, poultry, fish, or low-fat dairy products. The American Institute of Cancer Research calls this the New American Plate and recommends that you use it as a model as you begin eating smaller portions of meat and larger portions of vegetables, grains, beans, and other plant foods.

Thinking about your plate in this way will help you achieve your daily goal of eating five to nine servings of a variety of fruits and vegetables.

Getting these servings shouldn't be daunting if you understand portion sizes. Eat any one item listed below and you have eaten the equivalent of one serving.

> ◆ Meat: Not the
> Center of the Plate ◆
>
> In a primarily plant-based diet, meat does not play a big role. The New American Plate is two-thirds or more plant-based foods, so meat is a side dish. Experiment with stir-fry recipes, using meat as a flavor booster (try Mushroom-Asparagus Stir-Fry with Bay Scallops, page 189).
>
> Cancer experts recommend limiting meat intake to one 3-ounce (boneless, cooked weight) portion per day. That amounts to about the size of a deck of cards. Choose poultry or fish and limit red meat.

FRUITS AND VEGETABLES

FOODS THAT EQUAL ONE SERVING:

1 medium apple, banana, or orange

½ cup chopped cooked or canned
fruit

¾ cup fruit or vegetable juice

1 cup raw leafy vegetables

½ cup other vegetables (cooked
or raw)

Make those five to nine servings a day count by using the Top 10 "Super Foods" to meet your goal. Enjoy deep green cruciferous vegetables like broccoli, kale, collard greens, bok choy, and spinach. Add color to your plate with carotenoid-rich foods such as pumpkin, carrots, and tomatoes. Savor the rich sweetness of deeply colored fruits—strawberries and other berries, watermelon, and oranges. Try to eat most of your servings from whole fruits or vegetables rather than juices.

STARCHY AND PROTEIN-RICH PLANT FOODS

Starchy plant foods such as cereal, rice, or pasta and protein-rich plant foods such as beans also have a place on your plate.

FOODS THAT EQUAL ONE SERVING:

1 slice bread

1 ounce (about 1 cup) ready-to-eat
cereal

½ cup cooked cereal, rice, or pasta

½ cup cooked beans (dried or
canned)

1 medium sweet potato

½ cup corn, beets, or parsnips

When eating grain-based foods, go for whole grains. Choose grain products like bread, pasta, or cereal that list whole grain as the first ingredient. Whole grain foods not only provide more nutrition but they are rich in fiber. Fiber helps to speed elimination of potential cancer-causing compounds from the body, and it promotes a feeling of fullness that helps maintain a healthy weight.

FATS

As we've discussed, monounsaturated fats, essential fatty acids such as omega-3s, and polyunsaturated fats are important additions to a healthy diet. Good sources of these fats include olive and canola oils; cold-water fish such as salmon, sardines, trout, herring, and mackerel; nuts and seeds; avocados; and olives. Other sources of fat include dairy products like yogurt, milk, and cheese; choose low-fat varieties of these foods when possible.

FOODS THAT EQUAL ONE SERVING (5 GRAMS) OF FAT:

2 ounces lean meat (skinless chicken or turkey, pork, tuna)

1 ounce medium-fat meat (beef, 1 egg, skin-on chicken or turkey, fish)

5 ounces tofu

1 cup reduced-fat (2%) milk or cottage cheese

2 cups low-fat (1%) milk or cottage cheese

2 teaspoons salad dressing

1 teaspoon peanut butter

1 teaspoon oil, butter, margarine, or mayonnaise

⅛ avocado

12 peanuts

6 almonds or cashews

MAINTAINING A HEALTHY WEIGHT

Both the American Cancer Society and AICR guidelines for cancer survivors recommend nutrition and lifestyle goals that result in being as lean as possible without being underweight. In the United States, excess body weight is thought to contribute to as many as one out of five cancer-related deaths.

Excess body fat may promote and accelerate the development of cancer by:

• Causing the body to secrete more of certain hormones, including estrogen, which create an environment that is favorable to cancer development

• Becoming incorporated in cell membranes and changing them so that they lack the defenses they need to block entry of carcinogenic substances

• Decreasing the function of certain components of the immune system

Diabetes, heart disease, and hypertension are also linked to being overweight. When you're overweight, the extra fat cells make the body's tissues less sensitive to the effects of insulin, so your body produces increasing amounts of it. Too much insulin can lead to more rapid division of cells, and increased cell replication increases the risk that a random cell will mutate and lead to cancer. Maintaining a healthy weight can reduce the risk of insulin resistance, which is a risk factor for cancer and cancer recurrence. In one study, researchers gathered information from people in Europe over the course of thirteen years to explore how following AICR guidelines impacted risk of premature death from cancer. The findings? People who ate a plant-based diet and maintained a healthy weight had a 20 percent lower risk of premature death.

Identifying Your Calorie Goal

Here's a formula to help you determine a healthy calorie goal:

- Underweight adults: multiply your body weight (in pounds) by 18
- Normal-weight adults: multiply your body weight by 16
- Overweight adults: multiply your body weight by 14

You now have an estimate of the number of calories you need per day. For example, a 140-pound underweight adult needs about 2,520 calories a day. A 140-pound normal-weight adult needs about 2,240 calories a day. An overweight 140-pound adult needs about 1,960 calories a day. You'll consume more calories on some days and less on others. The idea is to average the target calories estimate. To help you track your daily intake of nutrients, including calories, fiber, sodium, fat, and protein, consider using mobile-device apps, computer programs, or websites like MyFitnessPal.com or LoseIt.com.

If you are in treatment, focus on getting the best nutrition possible. Eating a diet rich in fruits and vegetables has been shown to increase overall survival following cancer diagnosis and treatment. If you are obese or overweight, modest weight loss during treatment is not harmful if your treating oncologist approves, the weight loss is monitored closely, and it does not interfere with cancer treatment.

Here are some hints for maintaining a healthy weight: Make small changes for big results by filling two-thirds or more of your plate with plant-based foods and cutting back on foods that are calorie-dense (lots in small portions). Eat plant-based foods that are high in fiber; these foods will make you feel full longer and provide important nutrients. Practice portion control. For example, nuts are a healthy food, but a serving size is just ⅓ cup. Finally, get a personalized eating plan from a registered dietitian tailored to your eating style and particular goals.

Protecting Yourself Against Food-Borne Illnesses

Along with eating a balance of healthy foods, creating a healthier diet involves practicing food safety.

Food safety is particularly important for many cancer survivors, and especially for people in treatment. If you have a weakened immune system, your body is less effective at protecting you against illnesses carried by bacteria found in foods. Animal products in particular may contain harmful bacteria and other potentially dangerous pathogens. Remember, you cannot rely on your senses to determine if food is contaminated. Spoiled foods do not necessarily change in smell, taste, or appearance. Food can be unsafe to eat before it begins to smell.

The ACS offers general guidelines on food safety to help you and your family lower the risk of contracting food-borne illnesses:

• Keep all aspects of food preparation clean: wash hands before preparing any food, sanitize cutting boards and countertops, and scrub fruits and vegetables thoroughly.

• Use special care in handling raw meats, fish, poultry, and eggs.

- Thoroughly sanitize all utensils, countertops, cutting boards, and sponges that have come in contact with raw meat; keep raw meats and ready-to-eat foods separate.

- Cook foods to the proper temperatures: meat, poultry, and seafood doneness should be checked with a thermometer.

- Store foods promptly at low temperatures (below 40 degrees F) to minimize bacterial growth.

- Only drink pasteurized beverages; avoid fresh milk and juices.

- Avoid raw honey.

- When eating in restaurants, avoid foods that may have potential bacterial contamination, such as items from salad bars, sushi, and other raw or undercooked meat, fish, shellfish, poultry, or eggs.

- If there is any concern about water purity (e.g., well water), have it checked for bacterial content by contacting your local public health department.

- Wash hands thoroughly with soap before eating.

Shopping

Check the "sell by" and "best used by" dates on the product. The farther ahead the date is from the date you are shopping, the better. For fresh meat, poultry, and seafood, buy only if the "packaged on" date has today's or yesterday's date.

Buy only refrigerated eggs, and check for clean, un-cracked shells. When shopping, buy eggs, milk, meats, fish, and frozen foods last.

Storing

Store eggs in their original carton on the middle shelf of the refrigerator. Refrigerate or freeze meat, poultry, and fish as soon as you get home. Few food-borne bacteria can grow in the refrigerator, and none can grow in the freezer.

To prevent contamination, refrigerate leftovers within two hours after cooking or serving. Refer to the chart of the facing page for recommended storage times for keeping foods:

	IN REFRIGERATOR	IN FREEZER
Fresh meat	3 to 5 days	6 to 12 months
Hamburger	1 to 2 days	3 to 4 months
Fresh fish	1 to 2 days	2 to 3 months
Milk	5 days past carton date	1 month
Leftovers	1 to 2 days	2 to 3 months
Eggs	3 to 5 weeks	Do not freeze in shell

Preparing or Cooking

Avoid cross-contamination. Don't chop salad vegetables on a cutting board that you've just used to trim raw meat, poultry, or fish. Wash the cutting board, countertop, utensils, and your hands with hot, soapy water after contact with fresh meats. Change sponges and dish towels often.

Read the expiration dates on food products and look for signs of spoilage. Some food may be unsafe to eat even if it looks and smells fine. When in doubt, throw it out.

Be cautious about foods that may harbor unhealthy bacteria, such as soft cheeses and cold-smoked salmon. Soft cheeses include Brie, Camembert, feta, blue cheeses like Roquefort, and Mexican soft cheeses like queso blanco. Thoroughly reheat cold cuts, and cook hot dogs completely. Avoid eating alfalfa sprouts or the sprouts of other seeds; they may be contaminated with E. coli or salmonella bacteria.

Thaw frozen items in the microwave or refrigerator, not on the kitchen counter. Carefully rinse fruits and vegetables. Completely cook foods, using a food thermometer to ensure that meat is thoroughly cooked.

Before using eggs, make sure there are no visible cracks in the shell. Cook them until both the yolk and white are firm. Cook sauces, custards, or casseroles that contain eggs to at least 160 degrees F. Avoid eating foods that contain raw eggs, such as homemade Caesar dressing, ice cream, mayonnaise, and eggnog.

Cook meats until they reach the correct temperature: 160 degrees F for ground meats like hamburger, 165 degrees F for chicken and turkey—either whole or in pieces. Cook steaks and roasts to a temperature of 145 degrees F. Cook fish to 145 degrees F as well; the flesh will be opaque and flake easily. Foods like casseroles or leftovers should be heated to 165 degrees F. Use a meat thermometer, placed in the thickest part of the food, to test the temperature.

For cooking or heating foods in the microwave, be cautious about using plastic containers. Certain types of plastic, when heated, release compounds that may be harmful to human health. For example, some of these compounds can mimic the action of estrogen in the human body and may contribute to breast cancer and other hormone-sensitive cancers. To avoid this potential problem, use glass containers and microwave-safe lids to reheat your leftovers. Avoid letting any kind of plastic wrap touch the food.

Wrap and refrigerate leftovers within two hours—the sooner the better.

Safer Grilling

Animal foods, such as red meat, poultry, and fish, produce cancer-causing compounds when barbecued or cooked on hot stones. Called heterocyclic amines (HCAs), these compounds cause tumors in animals and may increase the risk of cancer in humans. Don't mothball your barbecue, however—there are steps you can take to minimize the formation of these compounds when you grill:

• Marinate meats before grilling to reduce HCAs. Use about ½ cup marinade for every 1 pound meat.

• Keep meat portions small for shorter grilling times.

• Trim the fat from meats; when it drips onto coals, polycyclic aromatic hydrocarbons (PCAs) are formed, which may cause cancer.

• Don't eat any charred or burned portions of meat.

• Grill fruits and vegetables, which do not produce HCAs.

COPING WITH POSSIBLE SIDE EFFECTS OF CANCER TREATMENT

CANCER, ITS TREATMENT, AND THE WORRY AND FEAR THAT ACCOMPANY the whole experience may result in some side effects that make eating more difficult and food less appealing.

Side effects vary from person to person and can even vary during different phases of treatment and recovery. (Some people don't experience any symptoms, or have just minor ones.) As a result, ways to overcome or minimize side effects also vary. What follows are some possible solutions; keep trying different approaches until you find the ones that work best for you.

It may be helpful to keep a journal of your symptoms and side effects. Use a little notebook or a journal app like iChemoDiary or Cancer.Net Mobile on your mobile device or computer.

Note what seems to trigger side effects, remedies that work and don't work, and questions to ask your doctor, nurse, or registered dietitian.

Be sure to keep your doctor informed about all side effects you are experiencing. Books, support groups, and the Internet may give you opportunities to discover and share tips and encouragement with other cancer survivors. And remember: Most side effects go away when the treatment comes to an end.

This chapter contains some tips for managing the most common treatment-related symptoms.

Nausea

- Call your doctor if you feel nauseated. It's better to treat the problem before vomiting begins.

- Keep track of when you experience nausea and its possible cause (time of day, foods eaten, events, surroundings). Share this information with your caregivers and medical staff.

- Ask your doctor or nurse about medication to help control nausea before and after treatments.

- Talk to your registered dietitian about ways to modify your diet to minimize symptoms.

- Ask family or friends to shop for groceries and cook for you if the sight or smell of food nauseates you. Stay out of the kitchen, or even leave the house, while meals are being prepared.

- Try cold foods, which tend to have fewer odors than hot foods.

- Experiment with foods and beverages that you have been able to tolerate when you've had the flu, morning sickness, or nausea caused by stress in the past.

- Listen to your body. Some people find that they need to avoid fatty, greasy, or fried foods; spicy, hot foods; foods with strong odors; or very sweet foods. Other people crave spicy foods and strong flavors.

- Avoid your favorite foods when you're feeling nauseated. You may develop a permanent dislike for them if you link them with feeling sick.

- Eat small meals slowly and frequently (every two to three hours).

- Rest, sitting up, for about an hour after every meal.

♦ For Nausea, Choose Foods Like These: ♦

* Clear liquids, flat soda, or ginger ale
* Frozen juice cubes
* Fruits or vegetables that are soft or bland (try pureed foods or jarred baby foods)
* Oatmeal
* Pretzels
* Sherbet or sorbet
* Skinned chicken (baked or broiled, not fried)
* Toast and crackers
* Yogurt

- Drink or sip cold beverages throughout the day, except at mealtimes. Ginger and peppermint teas may be soothing, and they're also good combined.

- Keep crackers beside your bed to nibble before getting up in the morning.

- Keep your mouth clean. Brush your teeth at least twice a day.

- If you're hospitalized, have the lids removed from your meals before the tray is brought into your room so most of the odors are dispersed in the hallway.

> **♦ Make Ginger Tea ♦**
>
> 1. Wash, peel, and chop a 1-inch piece of fresh ginger.
>
> 2. Boil the chopped ginger in about 3 cups water for 20 minutes.
>
> 3. Cool and drink the liquid. You may store the tea for up to 1 day, but if you have time, it's best made fresh each day.

- Ask your doctor or nurse about the use of acupressure bands on your wrists. They may help decrease your nausea.

- Wear loose-fitting clothing.

- Breathe fresh air, and try relaxation techniques such as meditation or listening to soothing music.

- Ginger (*Zingiber officinalis*) is an herb recognized to help with nausea associated with chemotherapy. Try drinking ginger tea or flat ginger ale. (If your blood-clotting ability is impaired while undergoing chemotherapy, check with your health care team before using this herb.)

VOMITING

- Call your doctor if vomiting continues for longer than half an hour.

- Wait an hour after vomiting stops before eating or drinking.

- Drink small amounts of clear liquids beginning one hour after vomiting has stopped. A teaspoon every ten minutes is a good place to start, then gradually increase to a tablespoon every twenty minutes, then 2 tablespoons every thirty minutes. Ginger tea, diluted juices, and clear broth are good choices.

- Begin with a liquid diet of teas and broths and gradually work up to a soft diet of applesauce, mashed potatoes, well-cooked vegetables, oatmeal, skinless chicken, fish, and rice.

CONSTIPATION

- Drink eight to ten glasses of liquid every day. Try keeping a bottle of water with you at all times. Add lemon, orange, or lime to the water to give it a refreshing flavor. You can also spike the water with fruit juice. Start with equal parts unsweetened fruit juice and water, and gradually make the mix with more water and less juice.

- Drink a warm beverage about half an hour before your usual time for a bowel movement. Try to drink it at about the same time every day to help your body establish a regular routine. Some people find that drinking warm lemon water or prune juice is helpful.

- Eat high-fiber foods such as raw fruits and vegetables, whole grains, and nuts. If you have trouble chewing raw fruits and vegetables, try grating or cooking them, skins and all.

- Add stewed prunes and raisins to your meals, or eat dried fruit as a snack.

- Add oat or wheat bran to dishes such as casseroles and homemade breads. Consuming 2 tablespoons of wheat bran a day will make your stools softer and easier to pass. However, because bran absorbs water, make sure you drink at least eight glasses of water a day.

- Use ground flaxseed, up to 3 tablespoons a day. Flaxseed is an excellent source of fiber and has a mild laxative effect. Grind the seeds in a coffee mill or blender, and then store the ground meal in a jar in the refrigerator or freezer. Sprinkle the meal on cereal, toss it on salads or with cooked vegetables, or stir it into soups. Flaxseed has a slightly nutty consistency but a neutral flavor. Start with 2 teaspoons of flaxseed meal and gradually add more.

- Try to move your bowels at your usual times. Many people find that after breakfast is a good time to try to have a bowel movement.

- Ask your doctor, nurse, or registered dietitian if you might need milk of magnesia or a magnesium supplement, a bowel regulator such as Metamucil or psyllium, a laxative or stool softener, or a combination of a laxative and stool softener.

- Take medications as instructed to prevent constipation.

- Get as much light exercise, such as walking, as your condition allows.

- Some pain medications can cause constipation. Talk to your doctor, nurse, or registered dietitian before this problem becomes serious.

DIARRHEA

- Call your doctor if you experience more than one episode of diarrhea each day or if diarrhea is persistent.

- Stick to a clear-liquid diet for twelve to fourteen hours after an acute bout of diarrhea.

- Increase your intake of liquids to six 8-ounce glasses per day unless your doctor or nurse has instructed you otherwise.

- Drink liquids between meals, not during meals.

- Consume plenty of liquids and foods that contain sodium and potassium. These minerals are often lost when you have diarrhea. Bouillon or fat-free broth, bananas, peach or apricot nectar, and boiled or mashed potatoes are good choices.

- Pass up beverages and foods that contain caffeine, such as coffee, strong tea, caffeinated sodas, alcohol, and chocolate.

- Avoid greasy foods.

- Stay away from foods with a high fiber content, such as fresh fruits, fresh vegetables, and whole grain cereals and breads.

> ◆ How to Use Herbs to Help with Diarrhea ◆
>
> Brew raspberry leaves as a tea, chew 3 tablespoons of dried blueberries, or make a drink by boiling crushed fresh blueberries in water for 10 minutes. Strain the fruit and drink. Avoid eating fresh blueberries; they may increase your diarrhea.

- Consume foods warm or at room temperature.

- Drink tea and eat applesauce, baby foods, flavored gelatin, and toast. Cheese and cottage cheese are also good choices, but first rule out lactose intolerance as the cause of the diarrhea. Foods that are easy to digest and produce fewer residues will give the colon a chance to rest and heal.

- Eat small amounts throughout the day, rather than large meals.

- Ask your doctor or nurse if you should use Immodium (an over-the-counter medicine) or a similar product to help manage loose stools).

- Try herbal approaches to diarrhea. Herbal experts recommend herbs high in tannins, like raspberry leaves and dried blueberries. The tannins in these fruits act as astringents to reduce intestinal inflammation.

SORE MOUTH OR THROAT

- Keep your mouth clean. Brush your teeth after eating and at bedtime. Use a soft-bristled narrow toothbrush and a sodium bicarbonate (baking soda) toothpaste with fluoride added. Dip the bristles in very warm water to make them softer. Floss your teeth at least once a day after brushing.

- Do not wear loose-fitting dentures.

- Do not use mouthwashes that have alcohol in them.

- Use cocoa butter, petroleum jelly, lip balm, or a water-based moisturizer to keep your lips moist. Do not use lemon and glycerin swabs.

- Try eating fresh or frozen watermelon. The high water content of the melon is very soothing.

◆ Try Honey for a Sore Throat ◆

A cancer support care study found that patients who swallowed honey before and after radiation treatment experienced significantly reduced oral mucositis (sore throat). Participants slowly swallowed 4 teaspoons (20 milliliters) of honey fifteen minutes before and after treatment, and then again six hours after treatment.

- Eat a well-balanced diet. Include foods that are high in protein, such as dairy products, poultry, meat, and fish.

- Choose soft foods:

  Applesauce, bananas, or canned fruits

  Cottage cheese

  Custards, puddings, and flavored gelatin

  Liquids

  Mashed potatoes, sweet potatoes, or macaroni and cheese (try Cottage-Style Macaroni and Cheese, page 209)

  Oatmeal or other cereals, cooked in nonfat or low-fat milk or

  soy milk for added protein (try Great Grains Breakfast Cereal, page 89)

  Peach, pear, and apricot nectars

  Pureed meats, tofu, or beans

  Scrambled eggs

  Soft or pureed vegetables

  Yogurt Protein Shake (page 86) or smoothies; tofu can be added to smoothies, or you can make tofu shakes

- Avoid irritating items such as citrus fruit or juice, spicy or salty foods, and hard, crunchy, dry foods (such as raw vegetables and toast), as well as alcohol and tobacco.

- Cook foods until they are soft and tender, then cut them into small pieces.

- Mix foods with low-fat yogurt, low-fat sour cream, or gravies and sauces made with broth and thickened with cornstarch. This will make them easier to swallow.

- Eat foods cold or at room temperature, rather than hot.

- Try tilting your head back or moving it forward while swallowing if you find that swallowing is difficult or painful.

- Drink plenty of fluids to avoid becoming dehydrated.

- Use a straw for drinking.

- Drink slippery elm tea or use slippery elm lozenges. The herb slippery elm is a mucilage (soft, moist, and viscous) that coats inflamed tissues.

• Try eating honey if you have a sore throat due to radiation treatment for oral or esophageal cancer.

• Rinse your mouth frequently during the day. Use a saltwater wash: add ½ to ¾ teaspoon salt to 1 quart water.

• Ask your doctor about anesthetic lozenges, sprays, or gargles that will numb your mouth and throat long enough for you to eat meals. Also, ask your doctor about using a mixture of equal parts viscous xylocaine, Maalox, and elixir of Benadryl or Gelclair to protect the inside of your mouth. These products require a prescription from your doctor.

• Do not hesitate to ask your doctor about a pain medication for your sore mouth.

LACTOSE INTOLERANCE

Lactose intolerance means that your body can't digest milk sugar—lactose—found in milk products. Symptoms of this condition may include gas, diarrhea, cramping, or nausea after consuming dairy products. To minimize symptoms, try the following:

• Experiment with getting protein and calcium from sources other than milk products. Soy milk, tofu, soy cheese, and soy yogurt are good substitutes for diary. Lactose-free or Lactaid-type milks such as acidophilus milk can often be consumed without causing symptoms.

• Use fermented or cultured reduced-fat milk products such as buttermilk, sour cream, and yogurt. They are often easier to digest than whole milk.

- Read labels carefully. Lactose is often used as a filler in products such as instant coffee and some medicines.

- Ask your doctor, nurse, or registered dietitian about pills for lactose intolerance.

- For many people, symptoms of lactose intolerance disappear a few weeks or months after treatment ends or when the intestine heals. Others will need to avoid dairy products indefinitely.

LOSS OF APPETITE

- Don't panic. Your appetite will come back when you're feeling better.

- Try to eat on a regular schedule and each time you feel hungry. Several small meals throughout the day may work better for you than three big meals. Even a few bites of food or sips of liquid every hour or so can help you get the protein and calories you need.

- Plan your largest meals for breakfast or lunch if, like many cancer patients, your appetite is better earlier in the day. Try dinner foods at breakfast time and breakfast foods at dinnertime.

- Drink plenty of fluids, even if you can't eat much, so you don't become dehydrated.

- Experiment with mixing fruit juice and soda water to stimulate your taste buds and give some variety to water and other fluids.

- Try to limit fluids right before eating; they may decrease your appetite.

> **♦ Patient Tip for Easing Canker Sores ♦**
>
> "I suffered terribly from canker sores before, during, and after chemotherapy. I found that the very best thing to put on the sore itself was Orabase paste. The paste sticks to the sore and covers it, acting like a bandage, and contains a numbing agent for pain. To help prevent the sores, I used toothpastes without sodium lauryl sulfate [an ingredient in most toothpastes], which can irritate the gums and lead to sores. I also tried to limit the amount of sugar I ate. The yeast produced from the excess sugars helped trigger my sores."
>
> **—MARIAN, CANCER SURVIVOR**

- Add variety to your menu: try new recipes and new ways of preparing old favorites, or eat in a restaurant occasionally.

- Arrange food attractively and create a pleasant environment. Eat with other people, if possible.

- Eat from a small plate with small portions; a large plate with large portions may seem overwhelming. When you're eating out, ask for an extra plate, and then spoon small portions onto it and eat from that. Or ask for a half portion.

- Don't hurry your meals. Relax and try to enjoy them.

- Talk to your doctor, nurse, or registered dietitian about your symptoms. They may suggest medications to stimulate your appetite, such as Megace or Marinol.

Loss of Weight

- Don't waste your appetite eating empty calories.

- Select high-protein, nutrient-rich foods if you're being encouraged to eat a lot of calories. Add coconut cream or silken tofu as well as a serving of protein powder to shakes and smoothies, spread peanut butter or almond butter on bread or waffles, snack on nuts like almonds or walnuts, and use avocado as a spread on a sandwich or toast. Add 2 teaspoons dry milk powder per cup of milk called for in recipes to increase protein and calories.

- Avoid drinking fluids before meals or filling up on soup or salad at the beginning of meals. Save your appetite for calorie-dense foods.

- Exercise about half an hour before meals to stimulate your appetite, but don't overdo it.

- Dine with friends or family members if possible. Most people eat more when they eat with other people than when they eat alone.

- Eat meals while you watch a favorite TV program or a great video. Distract your mind so you won't think about eating.

Weight Gain

- Remember that with some cancers, such as breast cancer, it's common for patients to gain weight during treatment. Be aware that there may be nothing you can do to control the weight gain. You may lose muscle mass, and this loss may lead to weight gain even though you aren't eating differently. To help manage your weight, focus on healthy eating and physical activity.

- Consume plenty of water—six to eight glasses a day.

- Drink warm fluids such as tea or soup about twenty minutes before meals.

- Try six small meals a day rather than three big ones.

- Eat regularly instead of waiting until you are too hungry.

- Choose more high-fiber foods: fruits, vegetables, beans, and whole grains.

- Keep a journal of what—and when—you eat. Use a mobile-device app or Web-based food-tracking program like MyFitnessPal.com or LoseIt.com. Notice when you are eating because you're stressed or bored rather than hungry.

- Fill a small plate rather than a large one, to create the illusion that you're eating more than you are.

- Get as much exercise as your condition allows.

- Consult with a registered dietitian for a personalized eating plan.

Changes in Sense of Taste

- Experiment to find which foods taste best. Many patients think that bland food is what they should be eating, but it's often the strong, spicy foods that sound and taste good. One patient even reported craving sauerkraut.

- Marinate meat, fish, and chicken to intensify the flavor.

- Choose moist foods like pasta and stews (try the Seattle Bouillabaisse on page 172).

- Use more or stronger seasonings such as garlic, onion, and ginger to add flavor.

- Eat tart foods, such as oranges or lemonade, which may have more taste.

- Try new and different foods. While some of your favorite foods may not taste as good for a while, there's a good chance that other foods, even some you haven't liked in the past, will be appealing. Discover new favorites.

- Eat chicken, turkey, eggs, or dairy products—foods that don't have strong odors—rather than beef and pork.

- Use plastic utensils if you're bothered by a metallic taste.

FATIGUE

Fatigue is the most common side effect of cancer treatment. Cancer-related fatigue feels different from other kinds of fatigue; it is often more severe, lasts longer, and isn't relieved by sleep. In a word, it can be overwhelming. Generally, cancer-related fatigue diminishes over time, but that may take up to a year. Talk with your health care provider about your fatigue; it may be due to a treatable condition such as anemia. We've compiled ten ideas for helping you cope with cancer-related fatigue:

- Power snack. Eating small meals or a snack every three to four hours will help keep your energy level constant. Try ¼ cup of nuts or seeds, whole grain crackers topped with 2 teaspoons of peanut butter, or 2 tablespoons of hummus as a dip with baby carrots to boost energy. Eat more when you're feeling well.

- Cut the caffeine. Caffeine-containing beverages and products—such as coffee, colas, and chocolate—can mask your fatigue. Instead, drink green or black tea. Tea has half the caffeine of coffee and is rich in cancer-fighting compounds called polyphenols.

- Fluids, fluids, fluids. Dehydration can add to cancer-related fatigue. Your body excretes approximately 3 quarts of water each day through perspiring, breathing, and urinating, and more if you exercise heavily. You can get approximately 1 quart of your water needs through food if you eat a diet rich in fruits and vegetables. The other 2 quarts (8 to 10 cups) should come from fluids, including pure water.

- Focus on whole foods. Stock your kitchen with fiber-rich whole foods, including fruits, vegetables, whole grains, and legumes. Whole foods provide optimum energy. Foods high in simple sugars—such as cookies, candies, and processed white flour—rob your body of vital nutrients that fuel energy processes. Use healthy convenience foods for quick meals and snacks: make a no-fuss salad with bagged organic greens, or use frozen vegetables for an easy stir-fry. Prepare and freeze meals ahead whenever possible. Label and date them before freezing.

- Keep moving. Physical activity can relieve stress that adds to cancer-related fatigue. Buddy up with a friend to take walks on a regular basis. Or break your activity goal into small, manageable segments: take a 10-minute walk at lunch, or use light-resistance weights or bands for spot strength training while you watch television.

- Accept help. Give yourself permission to let friends and family members help you. Prepare a list of tasks that friends can do so you can have them ready when they ask (see page 61 for some suggestions). Delegate heavy work. Arrange for a meal train, a personal chef, or a food delivery service. Use grocery delivery services and restaurant delivery in your area.

- Get organized. Spread your tasks over the week. Make a list when shopping, organized by store aisle. If you work, organize your clothes the night before.

- Keep it simple. Take a shower rather than a bath; it requires less energy. Use warm water rather than hot water because it conserves your body's energy. Use a terrycloth robe after a shower rather than towels. Bring your foot to your knee when putting on shoes so you don't need to lean over. Wear slip-on shoes. Wear button-down shirts rather than pullovers.

- Schedule naps. Take short rest breaks in the morning and afternoon, even if you don't feel tired. A 15- or 20-minute nap will boost energy. But balance your naps with adequate sleep and activity. Too much sleep can drain energy.

- Breathe and relax. Experiment with breathing exercises, stress-reduction techniques, or meditation if you're having trouble relaxing or sleeping. Try watching funny movies. Call Cancer Lifeline or a similar organization for information about relaxation and stress-management classes in your area. Check with your health care team for treatment options.

GETTING THE HELP YOU NEED

You may find that family and friends are eager to help, especially during the treatment process, but need some direction from you. On the other hand, maybe you don't have family or are physically distant from them, and you need to find out about other available resources. Here are a few suggestions.

Putting Friends and Family to Work

The next time someone asks if there's anything they can do to help, ask them to do one or two of the following tasks:

- Plan a week's worth of dinners.

- Accompany you to the grocery store.

- Take your list and go shopping for you.

- Help you prepare vegetables and other foods, or do it for you.

- Prepare a box of healthy, ready-to-eat snack foods.

- Organize friends and/or relatives to cook for you and your family. Each person might be responsible for making meals for one day. It works best if someone other than the cancer patient or caregiver organizes the effort. Meals should be either delivered in disposable containers or labeled so the containers can be returned easily.

> **♦ A Note to the Caregiver ♦**
>
> Keep a variety of foods available and offer them often. However, avoid urging food on cancer patients. They usually know they need to eat and are doing the best they can. What's more, eating may be the one area where they can exert some choice and control over their life.

- Run errands, such as going to the cleaners, library, or post office for you.

- Pitch in to help with household tasks, such as laundry, vacuuming, yard work, and taking out the garbage.

- Take care of returning phone calls, replying to emails, or arranging for bill payment.

- Pick up your kids after school and take them on an enjoyable outing.

- Give your caregiver some time off.

- Take you or your caregiver for a drive.

- Take you to a doctor's appointment.

- Listen.

EXPLORING RESOURCES

- Call an organization like Cancer Lifeline (1-800-255-5505; CancerLifeline.org) to find out about services and resources that are available in your community. Services often include transportation, support groups, meal deliveries, legal assistance, and financial aid. Contact your church, the nurse at your doctor's office, the social worker at the cancer center, or a community information line.

- Get connected. Use your computer for fact-finding and information gathering, and for linking up with support groups.

- Find a grocery store and some restaurants in your neighborhood that will deliver to your home. Order groceries online, if that service is available.

- Organize your kitchen so that foods are easy to find and within reach.

- Avoid buying food in hard-to-open containers or in cans if it's difficult to use a can opener.

- Stock up on readily accessible snack foods such as almonds, walnuts, fresh fruit, bean dips, refried beans and tortillas, string cheese, and yogurt.

- Keep ready-to-eat prepared foods on hand for when you're feeling under the weather.

- Turn off the ringer on your phone when you want to rest. Let your voice mail or answering machine take a message.

- Make an effort not to become isolated.

- Reward yourself regularly. Order some flowers along with your groceries, set up a "visit" with friends on Facebook or Skype, or get a massage—whatever will give you some pleasure.

- Find new ways to incorporate rest, relaxation, and exercise into your life. Each activity may last only a few minutes, but it will help to invigorate you.

HELPFUL WEBSITES

- **American Cancer Society (ACS)—Cancer.org**
  Provides information on ACS programs and events and local ACS chapters.

- **American Institute for Cancer Research (AICR)—AICR.org**
  The AICR is a national cancer organization specializing in the field of diet, nutrition, and cancer.

- **Cancer Care—CancerCare.org**
  Cancer Care is a national nonprofit organization whose mission is to provide free professional help to people with any type of cancer through counseling, education, information and referral, and direct financial assistance.

- **Cancer Hope Network—CancerHopeNetwork.org**
  The Cancer Hope Network provides support by matching cancer patients with trained volunteers who have themselves undergone a similar experience. Formerly known as CHEMOcare.

- The Cancer Survival Toolkit®—CancerAdvocacy.org/resources/cancer-survival-toolbox

  A free self-learning audio program to help cancer survivors learn how to communicate, find information, solve problems, and advocate. Developed by the National Coalition for Cancer Survivorship, the Association of Oncology Social Workers, and the Oncology Nursing Society.

- Caring Bridge—CaringBridge.org

  Caring Bridge offers online tools to set up a personal, protected site to stay connected with family and friends. One feature is a support planner calendar that helps loved ones coordinate care and organize helpful tasks. Similar organizations include: Lotsa Helping Hands (LotsaHelpingHands.com) and Share the Care (ShareTheCare.org).

- *CURE* magazine—CureToday.com

  CURE stands for "Cancer Updates, Research, and Education." A free quarterly magazine for cancer patients, survivors, and caregivers.

- Meal Train—MealTrain.com

  Meal Train provides an online platform to organize meals around significant life events. Some features include: a real-time meal calendar with the ability to customize dates, times, and meal preferences; invitations via e-mail and Facebook; and the ability to add booked dates to a personal calendar automatically.

- National Cancer Institute (NCI)—Cancer.gov

  The National Cancer Institute is responsible for conducting and supporting research on cancer. This website contains extensive information about the NCI and its programs. A valuable section of the site, called CancerNet, contains a wealth of information about cancer, treatment options, detection, prevention, genetics, supportive care, clinical trials, and a kids' page. There is also a Spanish-language site.

GETTING ORGANIZED

YOU AND YOUR FAMILY MAY HAVE DIFFICULTY FINDING THE TIME and energy to prepare healthy, nutritious snacks and meals, but eating right is undoubtedly more important now than ever before. The trick is to find ways to make shopping and food preparation as quick and easy as possible.

STOCKING UP

A good first step is to stock up on supplies that will make wholesome, healthy cooking and eating more convenient. Here are some suggestions for items that might come in handy.

Dry Storage

Vegetable bouillon or broth, low-sodium (powdered or canned)

Chicken bouillon or broth, low-fat, low-sodium (powdered or canned)

Canned beans and quick-cooking dried beans, such as split peas and lentils

Canned fruits in unsweetened juice, applesauce, dried fruit

Canned tomatoes, low-sodium (puree, paste, sauce)

Baking soda and aluminum-free baking powder

Cornstarch

Herbs, spices, and salt-free blends

Jarred spaghetti sauces, hot sauces, and teriyaki sauce

Low-sodium soy sauce and Worcestershire sauce

Vinegars (balsamic, rice, red, fruit, white)

Natural sweeteners like honey, malted grain syrups such as barley malt, molasses, pure maple syrup, Sucanat (unprocessed cane sugar)

Pasta (whole grain varieties, all shapes and sizes)
Sea vegetables such as nori or kombu
Soy milk
Water-packed canned fish such as salmon, tuna, sardines, or mackerel and canned chicken

Whole grain and white flours
Whole grains (brown rice, bulgur, barley, millet, quinoa, polenta, oatmeal, bran)
Whole grain pancake mixes

Refrigerator Storage

Milk and yogurt, nonfat or low-fat
Cottage cheese, ricotta cheese, mozzarella, and cream cheese, low-fat
Aged cheeses (Parmesan, Asiago, Romano)
Seasoned and plain tofu
Eggs
Spicy mustard
Salad dressings, low-fat

Extra-virgin olive oil
Fruits and vegetables, organic, seasonal, and locally grown when possible
Corn and whole wheat tortillas
Whole grain breads and muffins
Fresh salsa
Peanut butter and other nut butters (like almond or cashew)

Freezer Storage

Frozen vegetables
Frozen unsweetened fruit juice concentrates
Frozen fruits, especially berries
Boneless chicken breasts, lean beef or pork, and fish
Nuts (almonds, walnuts, Brazil nuts)
Seeds (pumpkin, sesame, sunflower)

Whole grain breads, bagels, waffles, and premade pizza crusts
Natural juice bars, sorbet, and low-fat frozen yogurt
Veggie burgers and soy-based sausages, hot dogs, and soy crumbles
Mozzarella cheese, part-skim

Handy Utensils and Equipment

Important Equipment

Sharp knives

Mixing bowls

Measuring cups and spoons

Steamer tray or basket

Nonstick skillet and bakeware

Salad spinner

Hand mixer

Blender

Nice, but Not Essential

Rice cooker (also excellent for
steaming vegetables)

Slow cooker (Crock-Pot)

Food processor

Microwave oven

Popcorn popper

Egg separator

Hand blender

Knife sharpener

Kitchen scale

Weekly Meal Planning

Make a goal to start creating menu plans. Start with a few favorite recipes from your collection and this cookbook and plan a week's worth of dinners. As you plan, keep your nutritional goals in mind. For example, "I want to have fish twice a week and meatless meals twice a week. I don't want to cook every night, so we'll go out one night and have leftovers at least once." Create a shopping list that includes all the items you'll need for the meals. By planning ahead, you can shop just once a week. Planning also reduces your chances of resorting to highly processed or fast foods when you're tired and hungry. These foods are often high in unhealthy fat, salt, and sugar and low in nutrients.

Don't expect to plunge right into writing weekly menus. Instead, you might want to make a commitment to plan one week of dinners this month. Next month, reuse the

> Every time you make a meal, snap a photo of it before you start eating. Post the photos on the fridge or online. Soon you'll have your very own food portfolio.

week of menus you've made and create one more. Soon you'll have numerous weekly menus from which to choose.

Save each week's meal plans on your computer or in a notebook or folder. Favorite plans can be reused when you're short on time or energy. Check websites and vegetarian and ethnic cookbooks for new recipes.

Examples of some meal plans follow. The starred (*) recipes are included in this book.

Menus

Menu 1

BREAKFAST: Whole Grain Pancakes*, fresh cantaloupe slices

LUNCH: Pita pocket stuffed with vegetables, drizzled with Cool As a Cucumber Dressing*

SNACK: Celery sticks stuffed with nut butter

DINNER: Seattle Bouillabaisse*

DESSERT: Pecan Honey-Baked Apples*

Menu 2

BREAKFAST: Yogurt Protein Shake*, Banana Bran Muffin*

LUNCH: Papaya, Shrimp, and Spinach Salad with Lime Vinaigrette*, whole grain roll, Simply Delicious Berries*

SNACK: Date Treats*

DINNER: Creamy Polenta and Bean Casserole*, Honey-Glazed Green Beans with Almonds*

DESSERT: Baked Custard*

Menu 3

BREAKFAST: Fresh fruit salad, whole grain bread topped with nut butter

LUNCH: Texas Black Bean Salad*, Chilled Avocado Soup*, rye or sesame seed crackers

SNACK: Low-fat string cheese, fresh grapes

DINNER: Spicy Miso Peanut Noodles*, Garlic-Sautéed Greens*

DESSERT: Very Berry Fruit Crisp*

Menu 4

BREAKFAST: Great Grains Breakfast Cereal* with berries

LUNCH: Crispy Mock Chicken Salad* on a whole grain bagel, carrot sticks and red pepper strips, pineapple chunks

SNACK: Lickety-Split Hummus*, whole grain crackers

DINNER: Grilled Chicken Skewers with Tangerine-Ginger Glaze*, organic baby greens with Zesty Tomato Dressing*

DESSERT: Almond-Crusted Pears in Orange Sauce*

Menu 5

BREAKFAST: Breakfast Burrito*, tomato juice

LUNCH: Basmati Rice with Lentils*, steamed broccoli, sliced kiwifruit

SNACK: Roasted nuts with fresh fruit

DINNER: Gingered Carrot Soup*, Ruby Chard with Garlic, Chile, and Lemon*, crusty whole grain roll

DESSERT: Raisin-Apple-Date Cookies*

SIMPLIFYING GROCERY SHOPPING

Planning ahead may seem like more work upfront, but when you know what you're looking for, your grocery shopping becomes easier and more efficient. What's more, you come home with foods you like that will contribute to your good health.

Getting the Most Out of Your Shopping Trips

- Keep a shopping list handy. Whenever you run out of an item, jot it down immediately. Keep the Top 10 "Super Foods" (page 9) in mind as you make your shopping list.

- Go to the grocery store once a week and buy only what's on your list.

- Get help from friends or family members.

- Shop at nonpeak hours that fit your schedule.

- Don't shop when you're hungry. Opt for a healthy snack before going to the store.

- During treatment or bouts of fatigue, consider ordering your groceries online, if that service is available in your area. Or find out if your grocery store offers local delivery.

Should You Buy Organic?

The evidence points to yes. Research has shown that people may be able to reduce or eliminate agricultural chemicals from their bodies by adopting an organic diet.

To guarantee that consumers get organic foods that are truly grown without synthetic pesticides, fertilizers, antibiotics, or sewage sludge, the US Department of Agriculture has enacted the USDA Organic Rule. When a food displays a USDA "certified organic" seal, this means that it has been grown free of pesticides and sludge, hormones, genetic modification, and germ-killing radiation. Organic meat and poultry means that animals have access to outdoors; are not given growth hormones, antibiotics, and other medications; are raised on 100 percent organic feed; and are not fed animal by-products. Organic milk comes from cows that have access to outdoors; are not given medications, hormones, or antibiotics; were given 100 percent organic feed for the previous twelve months; and got at least 30 percent of their diet from pasture during the primary growing season. There are no current standards for organic seafood.

If purchasing organic produce puts a strain on your food budget, learn what foods have the most pesticides and buy them organically grown whenever possible. The Environmental Working Group (EWG.org) publishes an annual list of the fruits and vegetables with the most and least pesticide residues. Examples of foods that consistently top the list of the "dirty dozen" include apples, bell peppers, celery, strawberries, and peaches. The "clean fifteen" produce includes asparagus, avocados, sweet corn, mushrooms, and sweet potatoes. You can find the most current complete lists at EWG.org/foodnews.

Read Food Labels Before You Buy

The labels on most packaged foods can steer you away from excess calories, too much sugar or sodium, and items that contain trans fats. Use food label information to help you stock your cupboards with more nutritious foods instead. Important things to look for include:

- **SERVING SIZE**: If you're going to eat the equivalent of two servings, remember to double the figures listed for calories and nutrients.
- **CALORIES**: "Low-calorie" means 40 calories or less.
- **TRANS FAT**: Avoid foods with trans fats. Words like "hydrogenated" or "partially hydrogenated" indicate trans fats in the product.
- **TOTAL FAT GRAMS**: All fats have 9 calories per gram. Carbohydrates and proteins have 4 calories per gram.
- **SODIUM CONTENT**: A healthy amount of sodium to consume is between 2,000 and 3,000 milligrams per day.
- **TOTAL CARBOHYDRATES**: Check the amount of sugar in the food. Remember that 4 grams of sugar equals 1 teaspoon. If a product has 32 grams of sugar, it contains about 8 teaspoons of sugar. To check the source of the sugar, look at the label.

You'll notice a column entitled "% Daily Value" on food labels. It is designed to tell you how much of a day's worth of fat, carbohydrates, and so forth the product contains. These numbers are based on a 2,000-calorie diet; your own intake may be higher or lower. Use them to give yourself a nutrient-value snapshot of the food.

For example, notice that the dietary fiber daily value (DV) for a 2,000-calorie diet is 25 grams. If a product has 3 grams of fiber, it has 4 percent of the daily requirement. Use this rule of thumb: If a food has 20 percent or more of the DV, consider that food to be high in the DV; low means no more than 5 percent.

It pays to be wary of claims on product packages such as "95 percent fat-free." Hot dogs, luncheon meats, frozen meals, and ice cream, to name just a few, often make these claims, but beware: These statements are probably referring to the fat percentage by weight rather than by calories. Fat-free products are not calorie-free, so be careful not to eat too much of them. Don't let the word "fat-free" give you a false sense of security.

You can trust the following key words, because they are defined and regulated by the government:

- **FAT-FREE**: Less than 0.5 grams of fat per serving (remember that fat-free products still contain calories).

- **LOW-FAT**: 3 grams of fat or less per serving (except for 2% reduced-fat milk, which has 5 grams per serving).

- **LEAN**: Less than 10 grams of fat, 4 grams of saturated fat, and 95 milligrams of cholesterol per serving.

- **EXTRA LEAN**: Less than 5 grams of fat, 2 grams of saturated fat, and 95 milligrams of cholesterol per serving.

- **LOW SODIUM**: 140 milligrams of sodium or less per serving.

- **VERY LOW SODIUM**: 35 milligrams of sodium or less per serving.

- **HIGH FIBER:** 5 grams of fiber or more per serving.

- **GOOD SOURCE OF FIBER:** 2.5 to 4.9 grams of fiber per serving.

Fat, Sugar, and Salt

Always review the list of ingredients on any packaged foods you buy. The most common food additives are saturated fat, sugar, and salt, so read the labels carefully to watch for these, which may be listed under several names.

Because solid fats are added to many processed foods, check the label for saturated fat content. Avoid products that have added trans fats (they are referred to as hydrogenated or partially hydrogenated oils). There is a direct, proven relationship between trans fats and increased heart disease.

Ingredient terms indicating sugar include corn syrup, molasses, honey, fructose, sucrose, dextrose, and fruit juice concentrate. Experts recommend limiting added sugars in processed foods to 25 grams (6 teaspoons) per day for women and 36 grams (9 teaspoons) per day for men.

Sodium content can also be extremely high in processed foods. Words for salt include sodium, sodium chloride, sodium bicarbonate, and monosodium glutamate. If you do eat some convenience foods, find ways to cut the sodium content. For example, if you are supplementing your meal plans with frozen, packaged dinners, try adding a bag of frozen vegetables to the entree: you will increase the number of servings, reduce calories and sodium, and get valuable added nutrients.

SIMPLIFYING MEAL PREPARATION

Here are some tips for making the cooking and cleanup processes as effortless as possible.

- Wash and cut up vegetables ahead of time and store in plastic bags in the front of the refrigerator. Use these for quick snacks and meals.

- Chop or mince twice as much onion, garlic, or ginger as a recipe calls for and store the rest in a resealable bag in the freezer for later use.

- Stop by the salad bar at the grocery store or pick up ready-to-eat vegetables for a stir-fry if your time or energy is limited.

- Cook a double batch of rice or beans to use as the core for recipes during the week. Reserve one day each week to cook batches of food.

- Double recipes and freeze half in individual serving-size containers.

- Keep prepackaged bags of salad greens or baby spinach handy, along with a supply of healthy convenience foods like canned or dry soups, canned chili, and crusty whole wheat breads for quick meals. These ready-to-go foods come in very handy when you're not feeling well enough to prepare meals.

- If friends or family members ask if there's anything they can do to help, consider suggesting that they bring a homemade dinner, prepare some ready-to-eat vegetables, or pick up a meal for you at the grocery store.

- Use quick and healthy cooking techniques such as these:

  - POACHING: Simmer foods in hot liquid just below the boiling point. No added fat is needed.

  - STEAMING: Place foods in a steamer basket over boiling water. This helps foods retain their water-soluble vitamins.

  - STIR-FRYING: Cook small, uniformly sized pieces of food in a nonstick wok or large skillet, using a small amount of oil, broth, wine, or water.

  - MICROWAVING: Use your microwave for defrosting, reheating, and steaming. But be cautious about using plastic containers for cooking or heating foods in the microwave. (For more details, see page 46.)

  - SLOW COOKER (CROCK-POT) COOKING: Dig that slow cooker out of your storage area. Slow-cooking is an easy way to cook batches of foods like beans and tough meats, since the cooking can be done overnight and the food is ready the next day.

  - GRILLING: Barbecuing is an easy and fun way to cook, but remember that animal foods such as red meat, poultry, and fish produce cancer-causing compounds when grilled. (For more details, see page 46.)

Choosing Fast Foods

When you don't have the time or energy to prepare meals from scratch, or at all, fast foods may be your best available option. Here are some tips for selecting the healthiest restaurant and supermarket fast foods.

At Restaurants

Become familiar with menu buzzwords. Ask how the dish is prepared if you are unsure, so that you will know what you're eating. Words that signal unhealthy foods include "fried," "hollandaise," "creamed," "breaded," "meat sauce," "Alfredo," and "tempura."

- Ask your waitperson about substitutions. For example, can you have a double order of vegetables instead of french fries with your meal? Can you have your ethnic dish served with fish or steamed tofu instead of beef or pork?

- Avoid fried items, and remove extra fat or skin from meat or poultry. Watch out for added fat from butter, sour cream, or creamy sauces. Try using flavored vinegar, salsa, low-sodium soy sauce, or fresh lemon juice on foods to enhance the taste.

- At fast-food restaurants, better options are to order a grilled chicken sandwich, single hamburger without cheese, salad, veggie burger, or vegetarian burrito.

- Select the salad bar to increase your intake of plant-based foods, but go easy on extras that are high in unhealthy fats, such as cheese, mayonnaise-based prepared salads, and bacon bits. Choose an olive oil–based salad dressing and nuts or sunflower seeds and olives as garnishes.

- Order water, iced tea, diet soda, or nonfat milk instead of alcohol, regular soda, a shake, or whole milk.

- Watch portion sizes. Portion "distortion" is common at restaurants. Order two appetizers as a dinner, or share an entrée with a friend. With supersized orders, ask your waitperson to bag the leftovers for your next day's lunch.

At the Grocery Store

Here are some guidelines for choosing from the dizzying array of foods in the freezer aisles.

- Select frozen meals that feature vegetables, such as Chinese-style veggies or veggie-and-rice bowls. If the vegetables are listed in the first few items of the ingredient list, you've found a good choice.

- Read labels carefully. Choose entrées that contain 15 grams of fat or less and no more than 500 to 800 milligrams of salt per serving. Cut back on products with a high content of sugar and sodium.

- Supplement the frozen meal with a bag of frozen vegetables or a bowl of salad greens.

- Select foods made with beans, including soy, and whole grains whenever possible.

Ideas for Quick-Fix Meals

Breakfast

Hot or cold whole grain cereal

Veggie omelet (add garlic, mushrooms, and red or green bell peppers)

Breakfast burrito—scrambled eggs with beans and cheese wrapped in a whole wheat tortilla

Whole grain toast topped with nut butter, such as peanut or almond, and all-fruit jam

Frozen whole grain waffle warmed in the toaster

Smoothie (try juice, yogurt or silken tofu, frozen berries, and flaxseed meal)

Lunch

Veggie pita pocket—toss chopped vegetables with canned tuna, salmon, or chicken; stuff in a whole wheat pita; and top with low-fat salad dressing

Grilled frozen veggie burger with tossed salad or a vegetable side dish

Baked potato topped with chopped vegetables, chili or salsa, and a sprinkle of low-fat cheese

Whole grain pasta with tomato sauce and steamed vegetables (try broccoli, zucchini, or your favorites)

Hummus with baby spinach stuffed in a whole wheat pita

Dinner

Stir-fried garden vegetables (fresh or frozen) with seasoned tofu or baby shrimp

Baked yams, sweet potatoes, or squash, topped with peanut sauce or cottage cheese

Pita pizza—whole grain pita topped with pizza sauce, lightly steamed veggies, and low-fat cheese, warmed under the broiler or in the microwave.

Burrito pronto—heat canned pinto beans, mash, and spread on a whole wheat tortilla; add shredded lettuce and salsa, then roll up and top with low-fat cheese

Noodle or rice casserole with chopped leafy greens (such as kale, broccoli, or spinach) and tuna or chicken

Bean supreme—mix two cans of your favorite beans, such as garbanzo and kidney, with a can of tomato sauce and make it spicy (add garlic) or hot (add chili pepper); heat and serve with a salad of baby greens

Snacks

Celery logs—fill celery sticks with an equal mixture of grated carrots, peanut butter, and crumbled mini shredded wheat

Banana sandwich—cut a peeled banana in half lengthwise, spread one side with nut butter (like peanut), and sandwich the two sides back together

Apricot treats—squeeze the edges of dried apricots to soften them and open them up, then fill each apricot half with a mixture of mashed banana, nut butter, and chopped nuts, rolled oats, or wheat germ

Apple and peanut butter—cut a medium apple in half, scoop out the seeds, and fill the holes with peanut butter

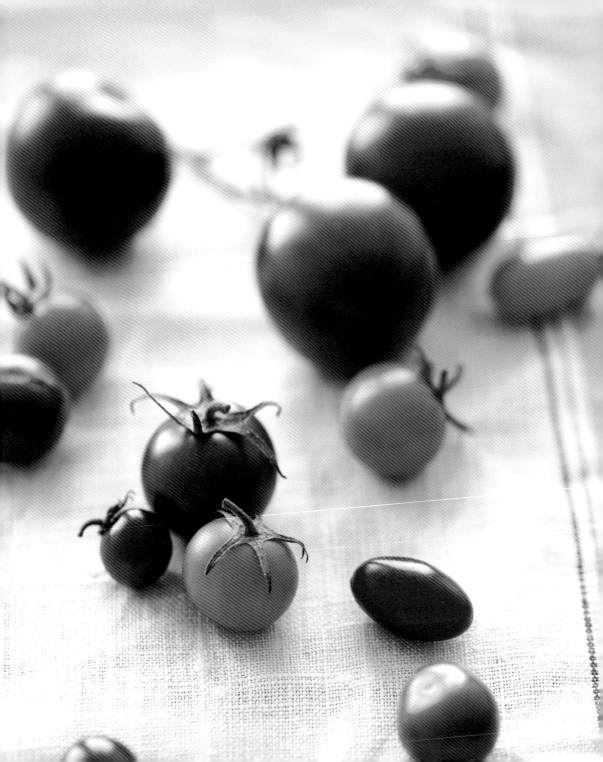

MAKING FAVORITE RECIPES HEALTHIER

RECIPE MAKEOVERS CAN TRANSFORM YOUR FAVORITE DISHES—WHICH may be high in fat, sodium, or sugar—into health-promoting meals. Here are some suggestions for simple, health-boosting recipe changes.

LOWER THE FAT CONTENT

- Cut the total fat in the recipe in half. For example, reduce ½ cup of olive oil to ¼ cup. Replace the fat with an equal amount of another liquid, such as broth, water, wine, buttermilk, or yogurt. Try substituting applesauce, mashed bananas, or pureed prunes for fat when you're making something sweet.

- Whenever possible, use vegetable protein such as beans, grains, legumes, and tofu, instead of animal protein. Begin thinking of meat as a condiment rather than the main course.

- Start using leaner cuts of meat. Packaging on lean cuts will include the word "loin" or "round"—such as top round or top loin. Use less red meat; substitute fish or skinless turkey or chicken breasts instead. Experiment with soy-based products, like soy crumbles, as a substitute for ground beef.

- Substitute evaporated skim milk in recipes calling for cream. Use nonfat or low-fat yogurt or sour cream instead of regular sour cream. Try low-fat or reduced-fat milk instead of whole milk. Low-fat buttermilk is also available and can be purchased in powdered form.

- Experiment with nonfat and low-fat dairy products, including cheese. Substitute strong-flavored cheeses like Parmesan or feta so you don't feel like you're missing out.

- Try steaming, broiling, baking, sautéing, or braising. When grilling, remember to marinate animal products to reduce the formation of cancer-causing compounds.

- Sauté foods in small amounts of olive oil and extend with broth, water, or wine.

LOWER THE SUGAR AND SALT CONTENT

Limiting your intake of sugar should be a priority. Highly sweetened and processed foods (like some colas, breakfast cereals, baked goods, and candies) can increase insulin response and promote weight gain—and they're full of low-nutrient calories to boot. Health experts also recommend that you keep your sodium intake under 2,400 milligrams per day (the amount in 6 grams of salt—a little more than 1 teaspoon). With that in mind, here are a few tips for decreasing sugar and salt in any recipe as well as some ideas for alternative seasonings that will up the flavor without negative health effects.

Sugar

- Cut all sugar measurements in half.

- Experiment with alternative sweeteners such as applesauce, blackstrap molasses, honey, prune puree, and fruit juice concentrate. Other sweetener options include rice and barley malt syrup, Sucanat, and date sugar; these can usually be found in the specialty section of large supermarkets or in health food stores. Note that because date sugar doesn't dissolve in liquid, it's not good in coffee, but it works well for baking.

- For every ¾ cup of liquid sweetener substituted for dry sweetener (honey instead of sugar, for example), decrease the amount of liquid in the recipe by ¼ cup, or add an extra ¼ cup of flour.

- Frost cakes while still warm with a thin powdered sugar glaze rather than a thick layer of frosting.

Salt

- Cut salt measurements in half. If a recipe calls for "salt to taste," add just a pinch and then taste. You can always add more if necessary.

- Skip or reduce the salt if a recipe calls for baking soda or baking powder. These ingredients already contain sodium.

- Get creative with herbs and other seasonings rather than relying on salt. Season vegetables with lemon juice, flavored vinegars, or your favorite low-fat salad dressing.

- Remember that most packaged spice mixes (taco, gravy, dressing, stew, spaghetti sauce) are extremely high in sodium and may contain unhealthy hydrogenated fats. Make your own spice blends, or purchase no-salt blends.

> ♦ **Making a Sandwich?** ♦
>
> Boost the nutrition power of your sandwich. Instead of using lettuce, try ½ cup of zesty broccoli sprouts or spinach leaves. Experiment with meatless sandwiches like pita bread stuffed with hummus and sliced vegetables as substitutes for ham or roast beef.

Alternative Seasoning Suggestions

- FRUITS: Caraway, cinnamon, cloves, ginger, mint, parsley, tarragon

- VEGETABLES: Basil, caraway, chives, dill, marjoram, mint, nutmeg, oregano, paprika, rosemary, savory, tarragon, thyme

- SALADS: Basil, chervil, chives, dill, marjoram, mint, oregano, parsley, tarragon, thyme

- PASTA: Basil, fennel, garlic, paprika, parsley, sage

- RICE: Marjoram, parsley, tarragon, thyme, turmeric

- BEEF: Bay leaf, chives, garlic, marjoram, savory

- LAMB: Garlic, marjoram, mint, oregano, rosemary, sage, savory

- **PORK:** Coriander, cumin, ginger, sage, thyme
- **POULTRY:** Garlic, oregano, rosemary, sage, savory
- **SEAFOOD:** Chervil, dill, fennel, parsley, tarragon

INCREASE THE FIBER CONTENT

- Choose whole grain rather than refined flours. You can substitute whole wheat pastry flour for any or all of the all-purpose white flour a recipe calls for. If you're incorporating other grains such as buckwheat, oats, or amaranth, do not substitute more than a quarter of the total flour called for.

- Try pasta products that combine whole wheat flour with white flour— you'll get the benefit of added fiber with a familiar pasta taste.

- Use brown rice rather than white, or try a mixture of half white and half brown. Experiment with other whole grains such as quinoa, millet, bulgur, and cornmeal, as suggested in our recipes.

- Try whole wheat or corn tortillas rather than flour tortillas for burritos, casseroles, quesadillas, and nachos.

- Add a colorful variety of fruits and vegetables to every meal, with emphasis on those in our list of Top 10 "Super Foods."

- Look for "100 percent whole wheat" when buying bread or baked goods. The word "whole" must come before the word "wheat," or you're not getting whole wheat. Don't be fooled by the words "wheat flour," "durum," or "semolina"—these are processed grains. Other grains, such as oats, corn, millet, and quinoa, do not have fiber removed when they are processed, so they don't need to have the word "whole" on the label.

Secrets to Recipe Success

- Change only one ingredient in a recipe at a time. That way, if your creation is less than a success, you'll know where the problem lies.

- Start out slowly. You can always further reduce fat, sugar, and salt after your taste buds have adjusted.

- Wait to announce the changes to family members until you've served the dish and it has received rave reviews or specific feedback.

- Accept progress without perfection. Every journey begins with the first step.

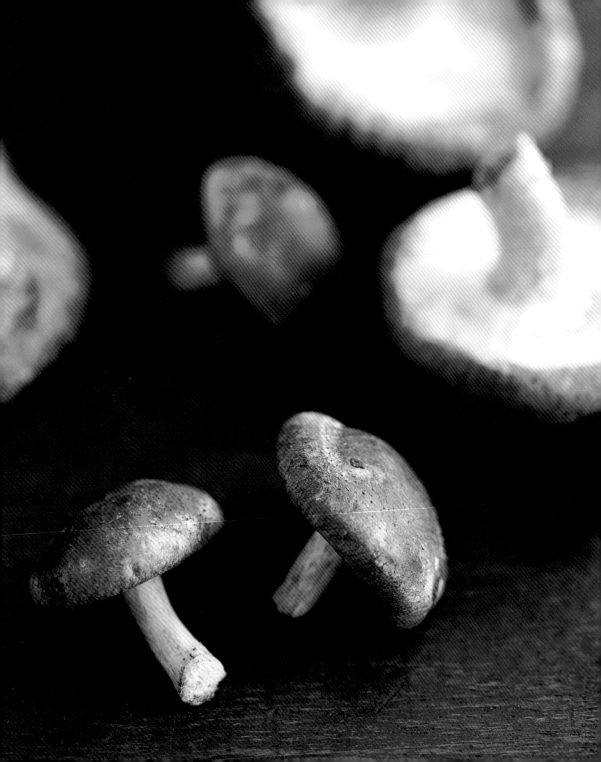

Breakfast

Yogurt Protein Shake 86

Great Grains Breakfast Cereal 89

Apple Muesli 90

Whole Grain Pancakes 91

Breakfast Burritos 92

Banana Bran Muffins 93

Blueberry Breakfast Cake 95

Applesauce Muffins 96

Oat and Date Scones 97

Savory Breakfast Strata with
Swiss Chard and Gruyère 99

Yogurt Protein Shake

A refreshing, high-protein shake loaded with vitamins, minerals, and fiber, great for breakfast or anytime. Using frozen fruit will make the drink thick, almost like an ice cream shake. Try this with any of your favorite berries.

MAKES 1 SERVING

½ cup nonfat or low-fat Greek yogurt
1½ teaspoons protein powder (made
  with whey, soy, or egg)
½ cup chopped fresh or frozen fruit,
  such as cherries, berries, peaches,
  or melon

1 banana, sliced
¼ cup or more fruit juice
1 or 2 pitted dates (optional)

• Combine all the ingredients in a blender, mixing until smooth. Add more fruit juice, if necessary, to reach the desired consistency.

PER SERVING: 294 calories, 3 g fat, 10 g protein, 65 g carbohydrates, 5 g fiber, 110 mg sodium

◆ Nutrition Tip ◆

Protein powders come from different sources, including whey, soy, and rice. Whey is derived from dairy sources, so avoid it if you have problems digesting those foods. Soy provides good-quality protein, equivalent to animal protein.

VARIATION: STRAWBERRY SHAKE

½ cup nonfat or low-fat strawberry
   Greek yogurt
½ cup frozen strawberries
½ cup apple juice

1 banana, sliced
1½ teaspoons protein powder
2 pitted dates (optional)

- Combine all the ingredients in a blender, mixing until smooth. Add more fruit juice, if necessary, to reach the desired consistency.

> **◆ Cooking Tip ◆**
>
> For variety, substitute vanilla-flavored soy milk for the yogurt or fruit juice. Add 2 ounces silken tofu for extra protein, carbohydrates, and fiber. Toss in about a dozen almonds for extra protein and calories.

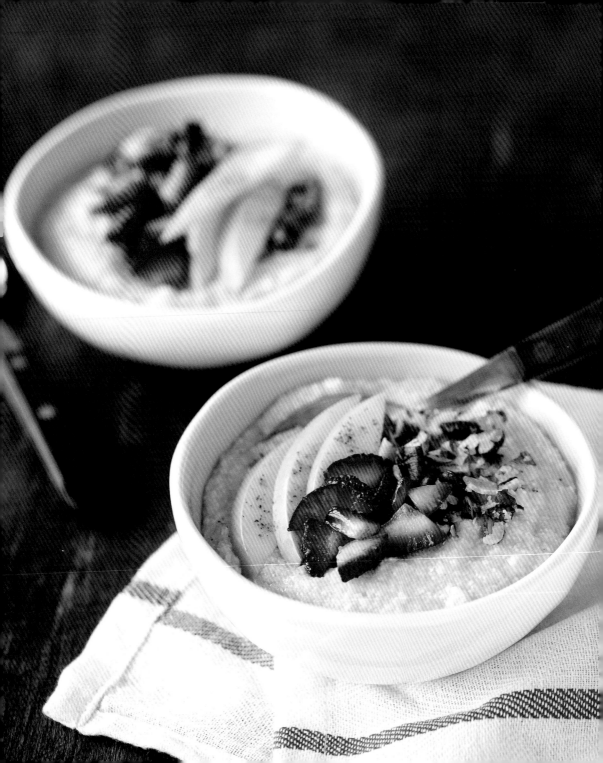

Great Grains Breakfast Cereal

Cooked whole grains are a good way to start your day. Add two or three tablespoons of chopped nuts to the cooked cereal, or swirl in a tablespoon of nut butter for added protein. For a breakfast express meal, make this cereal the night before and warm it up in the morning.

MAKES 4 SERVINGS

4 cups water

1 cup whole oats, buckwheat groats, or cornmeal

1 teaspoon vanilla extract

Seasonal fruit (berries, apples, pears, or other fruit), chopped

Soy milk, cow's milk, or nut milk

¼ cup nuts (such as almonds or walnuts), finely chopped

- In a medium saucepan, bring the water to a boil over medium heat. Add the grains and vanilla. Cook until the grains are tender but still well defined, 10 to 15 minutes.

- Remove from the heat, stir in the chopped fruit, and flavor with the milk. Spoon into bowls and top each serving with 1 tablespoon chopped nuts.

PER SERVING: 155 calories, 3 g fat, 7 g protein, 26 g carbohydrates, 4 g fiber, 582 mg sodium

Tip from Jeanne, a cancer survivor:
"I stir applesauce into hot cereal for an added flavor boost."

Apple Muesli

Muesli is a great comfort food that is easily digested and provides sustained energy. Fresh peaches, nectarines, or berries may be served alongside.

MAKES 4 SERVINGS

1½ cups old-fashioned rolled oats
1½ cups nonfat or low-fat milk
1½ tablespoons freshly squeezed
    lemon juice
2 Granny Smith or Fuji apples, cored
    and grated

¼ cup nuts (such as almonds or wal-
    nuts), finely chopped
1 tablespoon raisins
½ teaspoon ground cinnamon

- Combine the oats and milk in a large bowl. Let stand for 15 minutes.

- In a small bowl, sprinkle the lemon juice over the grated apple, then drain.

- Stir the apple into the oat mixture. Spoon into bowls and sprinkle with the nuts, raisins, and cinnamon.

PER SERVING: 239 calories, 7 g fat, 10 g protein, 38 g carbohydrates, 5 g fiber, 50 mg sodium

> **Tip from Maribeth, former Cancer Lifeline intern:** "I add ½ teaspoon of vanilla to the milk and drizzle ½ teaspoon of honey on top. To save time if I'm rushed in the morning, I use dried apple chunks."

Whole Grain Pancakes

These fiber-rich, versatile pancakes are a wonderful addition to your breakfast repertoire. This batter also makes great waffles—just reduce the milk to 1¼ cups.

MAKES 6 SERVINGS

2 cups whole wheat pastry flour
1 tablespoon baking powder
½ teaspoon kosher salt
1 tablespoon brown sugar, date sugar, or fruit juice concentrate

3 large eggs, separated, or 2 egg whites and 2 whole eggs, separated
2 cups nonfat buttermilk or soy milk
1 tablespoon butter or no-trans-fat margarine, melted

- Heat a lightly greased frying pan over medium-high heat.

- Sift together the flour, baking powder, and salt in a medium bowl. Set aside.

- In a large mixing bowl, beat together the sweetener, egg yolks, buttermilk, and melted butter. Mix in the dry ingredients until just moist.

> ♦ Cooking Tip ♦
>
> For variety, try using other whole grains such as oat bran, oat flour, amaranth flour, cornmeal, rolled oats, or buckwheat flour. Consider adding chopped fruit, nuts, or sunflower seeds to the batter.

- In a separate bowl, beat the egg whites to stiff peaks and gently fold them into the batter.

- Using a ¼-cup measure, drop the batter onto the hot frying pan, spacing the pancakes at least 2 inches apart. Cook until golden brown on each side.

PER SERVING: 225 calories, 5 g fat, 11 g protein, 36 g carbohydrates, 5 g fiber, 548 mg sodium

Breakfast Burritos

Breakfast burritos—scrambled eggs and beans wrapped in a tortilla and topped with salsa, sour cream, or plain yogurt—are a popular breakfast item at fast-food restaurants. Simple to make and delicious, this recipe provides a healthy alternative.

MAKES 4 SERVINGS

2 teaspoons extra-virgin olive oil
½ cup chopped onion
½ green or red bell pepper, chopped
2 cloves garlic, minced
½ teaspoon ground cumin
4 large eggs, beaten (or use 3 egg whites and 1 whole egg)

One 15-ounce can nonfat refried beans
4 whole wheat tortillas
½ cup plain nonfat yogurt or low-fat sour cream
Salsa

+ Preheat the oven to 350 degrees F.

+ In a large skillet, heat the oil over medium heat. Add the onion, bell pepper, and garlic. Sauté until tender. Add the cumin and remove from the heat.

+ Pour the beaten eggs over the vegetables. Return the skillet to medium heat and carefully stir until the eggs are soft and well scrambled.

+ Warm the beans in a small saucepan.

+ Wrap the tortillas in aluminum foil and warm them in the oven for about 10 minutes.

+ Fill each tortilla with a quarter of the eggs and beans. Top with yogurt or sour cream. Add salsa to taste. Roll up the tortillas, folding in the ends to form burritos. Serve immediately.

PER SERVING (1 burrito): 361 calories, 10 g fat, 20 g protein, 54 g carbohydrates, 12 g fiber, 623 mg sodium

Banana Bran Muffins

From Merrilee Buckley, former Cancer Lifeline intern

Most muffins are high in sugars and fat—not these fruit- and fiber-rich treats.

MAKES 10 MUFFINS

½ cup whole wheat pastry flour
½ cup unbleached all-purpose flour
¼ cup sugar
2½ teaspoons baking powder
½ teaspoon kosher salt
1 cup wheat bran

1 large egg, well beaten
1 ripe banana, mashed
¼ cup nonfat or low-fat milk
2 tablespoons canola oil
1½ teaspoons ground cinnamon
1 teaspoon vanilla extract

• Preheat the oven to 400 degrees F. Spray 10 muffin cups with nonstick cooking spray or line with paper baking cups.

• In a large mixing bowl, sift together the whole wheat and all-purpose flours, sugar, baking powder, and salt. Stir in the bran.

• Add the egg, banana, milk, oil, cinnamon, and vanilla and stir until just moist.

• Pour the batter into the prepared muffin pan, filling each cup halfway.

• Bake for 20 to 25 minutes, or until the muffins spring back when touched in the center. Remove from the pan and allow to cool.

PER SERVING (1 muffin): 125 calories, 4 g fat, 4 g protein, 21 g carbohydrates, 4 g fiber, 264 mg sodium

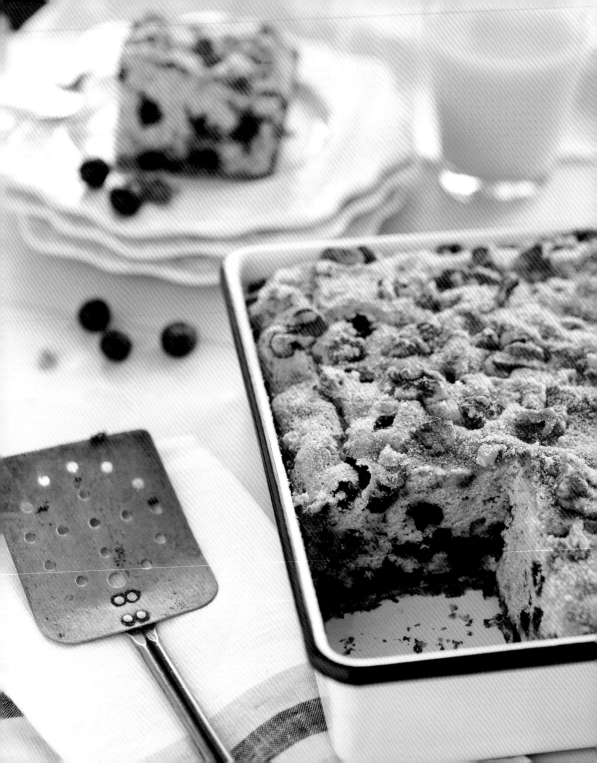

Blueberry Breakfast Cake

This breakfast favorite features blueberries, one of our Top 10 "Super Foods," in a rich, high-fiber blend of whole grain wheat and oat flours.

MAKES 9 SERVINGS

1 large egg
½ cup low-fat milk
½ cup plain nonfat yogurt
3 tablespoons butter or no-trans-fat margarine, melted
½ cup oat flour
1 cup whole wheat pastry flour
½ cup unbleached all-purpose flour
½ cup sugar

4 teaspoons baking powder
½ teaspoon kosher salt
1½ cups fresh or frozen unsweetened blueberries
Topping
3 tablespoons sugar
2 tablespoons finely chopped walnuts
¼ teaspoon ground cinnamon

- Preheat the oven to 400 degrees F. Coat an 8-inch square baking pan with nonstick cooking spray.

- In a large mixing bowl, whisk together the egg, milk, yogurt, and butter.

- In a separate bowl, mix the oat flour, whole wheat flour, all-purpose flour, sugar, baking powder, and salt.

> ◆ **Nutrition Tip** ◆
>
> Blueberries, both wild and cultivated, may be one of the richest sources of plant-derived antioxidants.

- Sift the dry ingredients into the wet ingredients. Stir the batter just to blend. Do not overbeat. Fold in the blueberries and transfer the batter to the prepared pan.

- For the topping, in a small bowl, stir together the sugar, walnuts, and cinnamon. Sprinkle over the batter.

- Bake for 20 to 25 minutes, or until the top is golden brown and a knife inserted into the center of the cake comes out clean.

- Cool on a rack for 10 minutes. Cut into 9 squares and serve warm.

PER SERVING: 214 calories, 4 g fat, 6 g protein, 40 g carbohydrates, 3 g fiber, 374 mg sodium

Applesauce Muffins

From Jean Warren, author of Super Snacks

These muffins use only natural sweeteners and make a wonderful breakfast or an easy lunch. Serve with yogurt and fresh fruit.

MAKES 12 MUFFINS

½ cup raisins
½ cup unsweetened apple juice
    concentrate
1 ripe banana, sliced
¼ cup canola oil
1 teaspoon vanilla extract
½ cup unsweetened applesauce

1 large egg
1 cup whole wheat flour
½ cup wheat germ
½ teaspoon baking powder
½ teaspoon baking soda
¼ teaspoon kosher salt
1 tablespoon ground cinnamon

• Preheat the oven to 400 degrees F. Spray a 12-cup muffin pan with nonstick cooking spray or line with paper baking cups.

• Heat the raisins and apple juice concentrate in a small saucepan over medium heat until the raisins are soft, about 3 minutes. Pour into a blender and puree.

• Add the banana, oil, vanilla, applesauce, and egg to the blender and puree.

• In a large mixing bowl, combine the flour, wheat germ, baking powder, baking soda, salt, and cinnamon and stir well.

• Add the wet ingredients to the dry ingredients and stir just until moist.

• Pour the batter into the prepared muffin tin, filling each cup halfway.

• Bake for 20 minutes, or until the muffins spring back when touched in the center. Remove from the pan and allow to cool.

PER SERVING (1 muffin): 193 calories, 6 g fat, 3 g protein, 22 g carbohydrates, 3 g fiber, 133 mg sodium

Oat and Date Scones

Scones are traditionally richer than regular biscuits due to the butter and egg. This recipe balances out that richness by being packed with fiber and whole grains, including oat flour.

MAKES 8 SCONES

1 cup unbleached all-purpose flour
½ cup whole wheat pastry flour
½ cup oat flour (place oatmeal in a blender and grind for 1 minute or so)
¼ cup brown sugar
2 teaspoons baking powder

½ teaspoon baking soda
½ cup (1 stick) butter or no-trans-fat margarine, cut into pieces
½ cup chopped dates
1 large egg, lightly beaten
½ cup low-fat buttermilk

- Preheat the oven to 375 degrees F.

- In a large mixing bowl, combine the all-purpose flour, whole wheat flour, oat flour, brown sugar, baking powder, and baking soda.

- Using a fork or a pastry cutter, blend in the butter until the mixture is crumbly. Stir in the dates.

- Add the egg and buttermilk, stirring with a fork until the dough holds together. Do not overmix.

> **♦ Cooking Tip ♦**
>
> A teaspoon of finely grated orange peel or ½ cup of dried apricots may be substituted for the dates.

- Gently knead the dough a few times on a lightly floured board. Add up to 2 tablespoons more flour if the dough seems too sticky to work with.

- Shape the dough into a flat 8-inch round. Cut into 8 wedges and arrange 2 inches apart on a nonstick baking sheet.

- Bake for 20 minutes, or until golden brown. Serve warm.

PER SERVING (1 scone): 234 calories, 8 g fat, 5 g protein, 37 g carbohydrates, 3 g fiber, 262 mg sodium

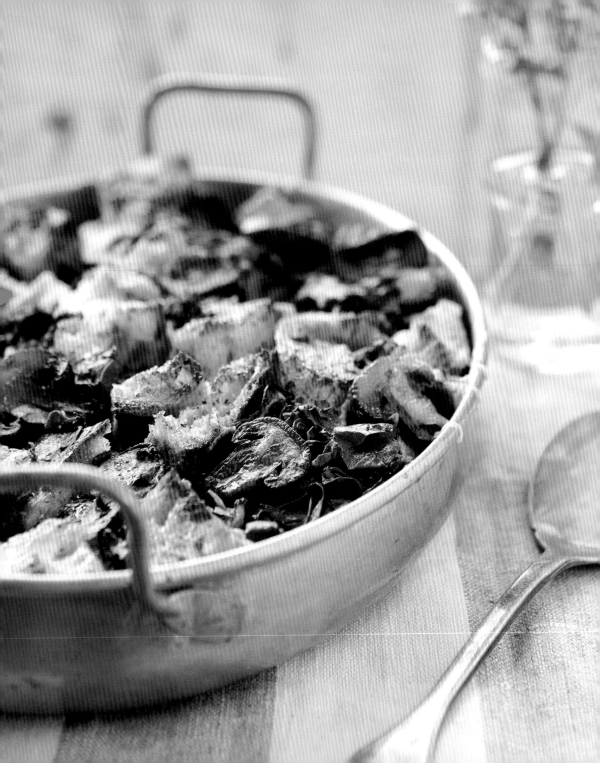

Savory Breakfast Strata with Swiss Chard and Gruyère

From Julie Hillers, cancer survivor

This savory dish of baked eggs combined with whole wheat bread cubes, Swiss chard, and Gruyère is a brunch hit. Serve any leftovers with our Spinach Salad with Poppy Seed Balsamic Vinaigrette, page 106, for a satisfying lunch. Note that this recipe requires at least an hour to prepare, and another hour for baking.

MAKES 6 SERVINGS

½ loaf (½ pound) whole wheat french bread, cut into 1-inch cubes (about 6 cups), divided
½ bunch rainbow chard or Swiss chard
1 tablespoon extra-virgin olive oil
1 clove garlic, minced

½ pound cremini mushrooms, chopped (about 2 cups)
½ cup (about 2 ounces) shredded Gruyère or Swiss cheese
6 large eggs
¾ cup milk
⅛ teaspoon freshly ground black pepper

- Spray an 8-inch square baking dish with nonstick cooking spray. Layer half of the bread cubes in the bottom of the dish until it is fully covered.

- Wash the chard and pat dry. Remove the stems and chop into ½-inch pieces. Cut the leaves into 2-inch pieces. You should have about 4 cups of chopped chard.

- In a large frying pan, heat the oil over medium heat, and add the chopped chard stems. Cook for 2 minutes, or until tender. Add the chard leaves and garlic and cook for another 3 to 4 minutes, or until the leaves are wilted. Layer the chard over the bread cubes in the baking dish.

- Put the mushrooms in the same frying pan and sauté for about 5 minutes, or until lightly browned and soft.

continued

- Layer the mushrooms over the chard, and then sprinkle with the shredded cheese. Layer the remaining bread cubes over the top.

- In a large bowl, beat the eggs and milk with a fork. Add the pepper, and then pour the mixture evenly over the bread cubes.

- Cover the dish and refrigerate for at least 1 hour or preferably overnight.

- Preheat the oven to 375 degrees F.

- Bake the strata, uncovered, for 55 to 60 minutes, or until a knife inserted 1 inch from the center comes out clean. Remove from oven and let stand for 5 minutes before serving.

PER SERVING: 230 calories, 7 g fat, 14 g protein, 28 g carbohydrates, 2 g fiber, 430 mg sodium

Salads and Appetizers

Papaya, Shrimp, and Spinach Salad with Lime Vinaigrette

From Chef Kathy Casey, cookbook author

An easy-to-prepare salad, this dish has a medley of colors and flavors.

MAKES 6 SERVINGS

1 head butter lettuce
1 bunch fresh spinach
1 large, firm-ripe papaya, peeled, seeded, and diced
1 large orange, peeled and diced

1 large, ripe avocado, peeled, pitted, and diced
½ cup sliced almonds, lightly toasted
½ pound cooked bay shrimp (optional)
½ cup Lime Vinaigrette (recipe follows)

- Wash and dry the lettuce and spinach, and cut or tear into bite-size pieces. Place in a large bowl and add the diced papaya, orange, avocado, almonds, and shrimp.

- Drizzle in some of the Lime Vinaigrette and toss gently to coat the salad evenly.

- Serve immediately, passing the remaining vinaigrette at the table.

PER SERVING: 314 calories, 21 g fat, 14 g protein, 21 g carbohydrates, 7 g fiber, 384 mg sodium

> ◆ Chef's Note ◆
>
> This salad is also great as an entrée, topped with grilled prawns instead of bay shrimp.

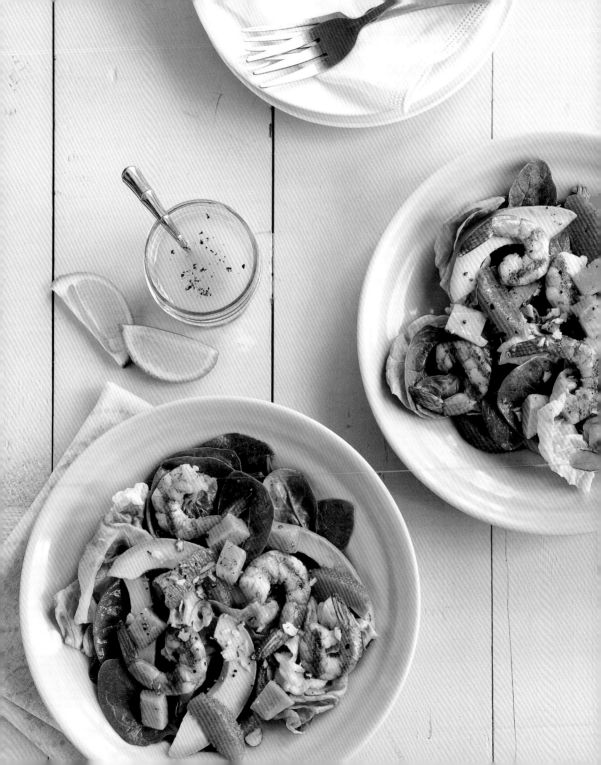

LIME VINAIGRETTE

MAKES ¾ CUP

¼ cup lime marmalade
  (preferably Rose's)
Juice of 2 medium limes (about
  ¼ cup)
2 teaspoons orange juice concentrate

½ teaspoon Dijon mustard
½ teaspoon kosher salt
½ teaspoon ground coriander
⅛ teaspoon cayenne pepper
⅓ cup canola oil

- Place the lime marmalade in a medium bowl and stir until the lumps are dissolved.

- Add the lime juice and whisk until smooth. Stir in the orange juice concentrate, mustard, salt, coriander, and cayenne.

- Slowly whisk in the oil until the dressing is smooth and emulsified.

PER SERVING (2 tablespoons): 140 calories, 13 g fat, 0 g protein, 8 g carbohydrates, 0 g fiber, 209 mg sodium

Crunchy Broccoli and Carrot Salad

From Mary Mataja, cancer survivor

This bold, crunchy salad is tangy-sweet with vibrant colors and flavors. Leftovers will keep well for several days to provide handy lunches or snacks.

MAKES 16 SERVINGS

3 broccoli crowns with stems
1½ cups shredded carrots
4 green onions, sliced
½ cup raisins
¼ cup dried cranberries

¼ cup low-fat mayonnaise
⅓ cup rice vinegar
¼ teaspoon freshly ground black
  pepper

- Break the broccoli crowns into florets and cut the stems into ½-inch or smaller pieces (if they are too large, they won't absorb the dressing well). You should have about 6 cups chopped broccoli.

- Put the broccoli, carrots, green onions, raisins, and cranberries in a large bowl and mix well.

- Whisk the mayonnaise, rice vinegar, and pepper in a small bowl. Pour the dressing over the broccoli mixture and toss to coat.

- Let the salad stand for at least 30 minutes, or overnight, before serving. Store any leftover salad in a resealable container in the refrigerator for several days.

PER SERVING (½ cup): 40 calories, 1 g fat, 1 g protein, 8 g carbohydrates, 1 g fiber, 40 mg sodium

♦ Contributor Tip ♦

Twist broccoli florets off the stalk near the neck of the floret. You can then snap the crowns off in small pieces. If you are serving this salad the next day and it seems a little dry, just splash with additional rice vinegar.

Spinach Salad with Poppy Seed Balsamic Vinaigrette

A special dressing makes this spinach salad stand out from the crowd. In spring and summer, add fresh strawberries. In autumn and winter, try dried apricots.

MAKES 4 SERVINGS

1 tablespoon poppy seeds
1 tablespoon sesame seeds
2 tablespoons sugar
¼ cup balsamic vinegar
2 tablespoons extra-virgin olive oil
3 tablespoons grape or apple juice
    (grape adds a nice flavor)

½ teaspoon Worcestershire sauce
½ teaspoon paprika
2 bunches spinach
½ cup walnuts or hazelnuts, chopped
2 tablespoons chopped green onion,
    for garnish (optional)

- To make the poppy seed dressing, in a small bowl, whisk together the poppy and sesame seeds, sugar, balsamic vinegar, oil, juice, Worcestershire, and paprika.

- To assemble the salad, wash the spinach and tear it into bite-size pieces (you should have about 4 cups). Put into a large salad bowl. Pour the vinaigrette over the spinach. Toss the salad and top with the nuts and green onion.

PER SERVING: 143 calories, 9 g fat, 3 g protein, 15 g carbohydrates, 2 g fiber, 55 mg sodium

Avocado-Dressed Fresh Kale Salad

From Mary Mataja, cancer survivor

Enjoy the vital flavors of raw kale paired with sweet corn and avocado. Use in-season corn if possible as it's sweeter and has a nice texture, though frozen corn will work too. Prepared with the help of a food processor, this recipe is grown-up food that's fun to make—you'll be getting your hands dirty with this one.

MAKES 6 SERVINGS

1 bunch fresh dill
1 red or sweet onion
2 cloves garlic
1 bunch raw kale (any variety)
1 red bell pepper, seeded and diced (about 1 cup)
1 large or 2 small roma tomatoes, diced (about 1 cup)

Kernels from 2 to 3 ears corn, or 2 to 3 cups thawed frozen corn
Juice of 1 lemon (about 3 tablespoons)
3 tablespoons balsamic vinegar
2 tablespoons extra-virgin olive oil
1 to 2 medium ripe avocados

- Pulse the dill in a food processor until finely chopped, then transfer to a large bowl. Pulse the onion and garlic until finely chopped and transfer to the bowl. Pulse the kale, in 2 or 3 batches as needed, until finely chopped and transfer to the bowl.

- Add the bell pepper, tomato, and corn to the bowl.

- In a small bowl, whisk together the lemon juice, balsamic vinegar, and oil. Pour over the vegetables and toss.

- Scoop the avocados into the bowl. Using clean hands, mash all the ingredients together. The avocados should be "absorbed" into the salad.

- Cover and refrigerate for at least 1 hour, or overnight, before serving. The salad keeps well for 3 to 4 days in the refrigerator.

PER SERVING (1 cup): 270 calories, 15 g fat, 6 g protein, 32 g carbohydrates, 9 g fiber, 230 mg sodium

Texas Black Bean Salad

Rich black beans, crunchy corn, and a hint of chili make this a perfect dinner or side dish. Make a large batch and freeze extra servings for later.

MAKES 8 SERVINGS

Two 15-ounce cans low-sodium black beans (about 3 cups), drained

1 cup diced sweet onion (½ medium onion)

1 cup diced red bell pepper (½ large pepper)

1 cup diced green bell pepper (½ large pepper)

2 cups fresh or thawed frozen organic corn

¼ cup chopped fresh cilantro or parsley

Juice from 2 limes (about ¼ cup)

2 tablespoons extra-virgin olive oil

1½ to 2 teaspoons chili powder

½ to 1 teaspoon ground cumin

½ teaspoon dried oregano

Dash of cayenne pepper

Freshly ground black pepper

- Put the black beans, onion, red and green peppers, corn, and cilantro in a large bowl and mix well.

- In a small bowl, whisk together the lime juice, oil, chili powder, cumin, oregano, cayenne, and black pepper.

- Pour the dressing over the bean salad and stir well. Refrigerate for at least 2 hours before serving.

PER SERVING (1 cup): 185 calories, 9 g fat, 5 g protein, 30 g carbohydrates, 9 g fiber, 434 mg sodium

> **♦ Nutrition Tip ♦**
>
> Legumes, like black beans, are richer in high-quality protein than most other plant foods.

Crispy Mock Chicken Salad

With a hint of curry and the sweetness of raisins, this tasty spread can be a topping for mixed greens or stuffed inside a whole wheat pita.

MAKES 4 SERVINGS

2 tablespoons canola or coconut oil
One 8-ounce package tempeh,
   crumbled
1 cup chopped celery
½ cup chopped carrot
½ cup minced fresh parsley
2 tablespoons finely diced red or
   yellow onion

½ cup low-fat mayonnaise
¼ cup raw cashews
1 tablespoon currants or raisins
1 teaspoon curry powder
Kosher salt and freshly ground black
   pepper

- Heat the oil in a large heavy pan over medium-high heat. Add the crumbled tempeh to the pan and cook for 3 to 4 minutes, or until crispy and golden brown.

- Transfer the tempeh to a large bowl and stir in the remaining ingredients. Season to taste with salt and pepper.

PER SERVING (1 cup): 430 calories, 32 g fat, 17 g protein, 25 g carbohydrates, 3 g fiber, 290 mg sodium

♦ Nutrition Note ♦

A traditional Indonesian food developed over five centuries ago, tempeh is a fermented food made from soy beans. Fermented foods are a rich source of gut-friendly bacteria that stimulate the immune system.

Waldorf Salad

Enjoy the delightful combination of textures in this healthy update of the classic salad.

MAKES 6 TO 8 SERVINGS

¾ cup plain nonfat yogurt
¼ cup low-fat sour cream
¼ cup low-fat mayonnaise
Juice from 1 medium orange
   (about ¼ cup)
¼ teaspoon ground nutmeg
2 Red or Golden Delicious apples,
   cored and chopped

2 Fuji or Granny Smith apples, cored
   and chopped
2 stalks celery, chopped
1 cup red or green seedless grapes
½ cup walnuts, chopped
½ cup raisins
4 to 6 cups salad greens

- To make the dressing, in a small bowl, whisk together the yogurt, sour cream, mayonnaise, orange juice, and nutmeg.

- To assemble the salad, in a medium bowl, combine the apples, celery, grapes, walnuts, and raisins.

- Toss the dressing with the apple mixture. Chill.

- Serve the salad on a bed of greens.

PER SERVING: 205 calories, 8 g fat, 5 g protein, 32 g carbohydrates, 3 g fiber, 80 mg sodium

> **• Nutrition Tip •**
>
> Walnuts are a plant source of immunity-boosting omega-3 fatty acids and, like all nuts, are also rich in protein.

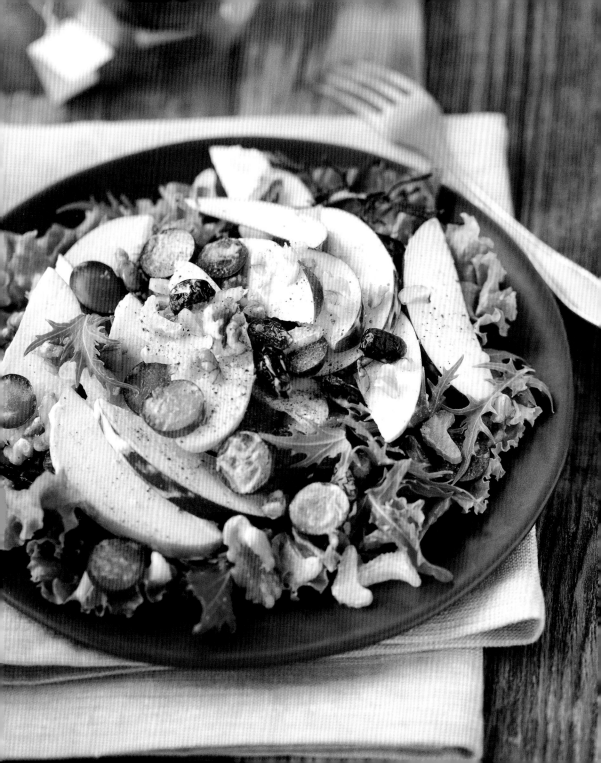

Zesty Tomato Dressing

A delicious alternative to traditional vinaigrettes, this dressing adds a splash of color to salads.

MAKES 8 SERVINGS

½ cup tomato juice
1 tablespoon extra-virgin olive oil
Juice from ½ small lemon (about
   1 tablespoon)
1 tablespoon vinegar

¼ teaspoon dry mustard, or 1 teaspoon Dijon mustard
1 tablespoon finely chopped onion
1 teaspoon finely chopped parsley

♦ Combine all the ingredients and mix until well blended.

PER SERVING: 20 calories, 2 g fat, 0 g protein, 1 g carbohydrates, 0 g fiber, 54 mg sodium

Cool as a Cucumber Dressing

A simple, high-protein recipe for salad dressing or vegetable dip. Stuff pita bread with fresh vegetables and drizzle this creamy dressing over the top.

MAKES 2½ CUPS

1½ cups plain nonfat yogurt with live
   cultures (see Nutrition Note)
½ cup low-fat sour cream
2 cloves garlic, crushed
Juice from 1 lemon (about
   2 tablespoons)

2 tablespoons chopped fresh dill
½ medium cucumber, very finely
   grated
¼ cup walnuts, chopped

• Blend together all the ingredients in a medium mixing bowl. Refrigerate until ready to serve.

PER SERVING (1 tablespoon): 15 calories, 1 g fat, 1 g protein, 1 g carbohydrates, 0 g fiber, 8 mg sodium

> ♦ **Nutrition Note** ♦
>
> Yogurt can often be consumed by people who are lactose intolerant. Because yogurt with active cultures is predigested, the amount of milk sugars is very low.

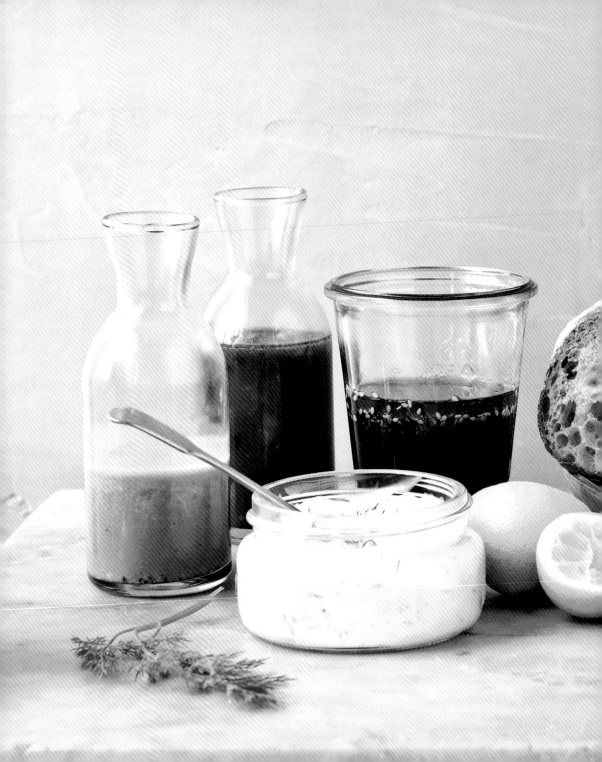

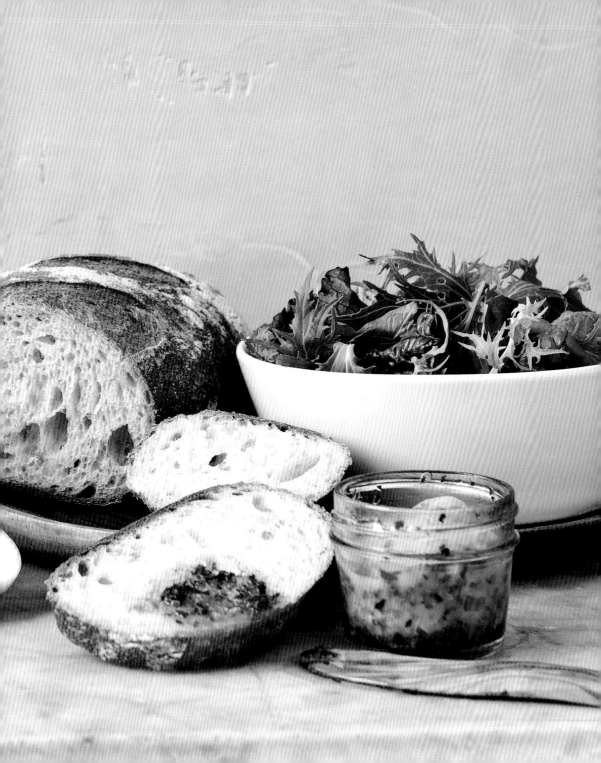

Olive Oil and Herb Spread

This mixture is a healthy alternative to butter or margarine. Keep it in your freezer as a handy and tasty spread for bread.

MAKES ½ CUP

½ cup extra-virgin olive oil
1 tablespoon dried or 2 tablespoons
    fresh basil, oregano, rosemary,
    crushed red pepper flakes, or
    minced garlic

- In a small bowl, mix the oil with the seasonings of your choice.

- Pour the mixture into a cruet and place in the freezer. Store in the freezer between uses. (Let sit at room temperature to regain spreadable consistency.)

PER SERVING (1 tablespoon): 120 calories, 14 g fat, 0 g protein, 0 g carbohydrates, 0 g fiber, 0 mg sodium

Creamy Artichoke Dip

From Bharti Kirchner, author of The Bold Vegetarian

This quick and easy recipe can be used as a dip or drizzled on top of your favorite salad. Don't replace the honey mustard with another type of mustard—the flavor will be off.

MAKES 1¼ CUPS

One 6.5-ounce jar artichoke hearts, including liquid

1 tablespoon extra-virgin olive oil

1 tablespoon rice vinegar or white wine vinegar

1 tablespoon or more honey mustard

Salt

- Put the artichoke hearts with liquid, oil, vinegar, and honey mustard in a blender. Blend until creamy. Add more honey mustard if desired, mixing in 1 teaspoon at a time with a spoon. Season to taste with salt.

PER SERVING (2 tablespoons): 25 calories, 1.5 g fat, 1 g protein, 3 g carbohydrates, 0 g fiber, 125 mg sodium

Lickety-Split Hummus

Homemade hummus is quick and easy to make. Use this versatile food as a dip for vegetables, as a sandwich filling, or as a spread on whole grain crackers.

MAKES 16 SERVINGS

2 or more cloves garlic, smashed
2 tablespoons extra-virgin olive oil
1 tablespoon tahini
Juice from 1 lemon (about
  2 tablespoons)

One 15-ounce can organic garbanzo
  beans
½ teaspoon kosher or sea salt
2 tablespoons water

• Put the garlic in a blender or food processor with the oil, tahini, and lemon juice. Blend until smooth.

• Add the garbanzo beans and salt and blend. Add the water and blend for 5 minutes. For a thinner consistency, add more water.

PER SERVING: 52 calories, 3 g fat, 2 g protein, 5 g carbohydrates, 1 g fiber, 72 mg sodium

Tip from Jenn, who perfected this recipe:
"Adding water gives the hummus just the right consistency. I start with 2 tablespoons, then add more until I get the smoothness I want."

Tropical Salsa

Pair this unique salsa with baked tortilla chips for a fun way to eat fruits.

MAKES 16 SERVINGS

1 mango, peeled, pitted, and diced
1 pint fresh strawberries, diced
½ fresh pineapple, peeled and diced
3 kiwis, peeled and diced

Juice from 1 lime (about 2
   tablespoons)
2 tablespoons chopped cilantro
1 serrano chile pepper, minced
   (optional)

• Place all the ingredients in a medium bowl and mix well. Plan to use this salsa within a day; it does not keep well.

PER SERVING (2 tablespoons): 20 calories, .11 g fat, .35 g protein, 4 g carbohydrates, .71 g fiber, 1.75 mg sodium

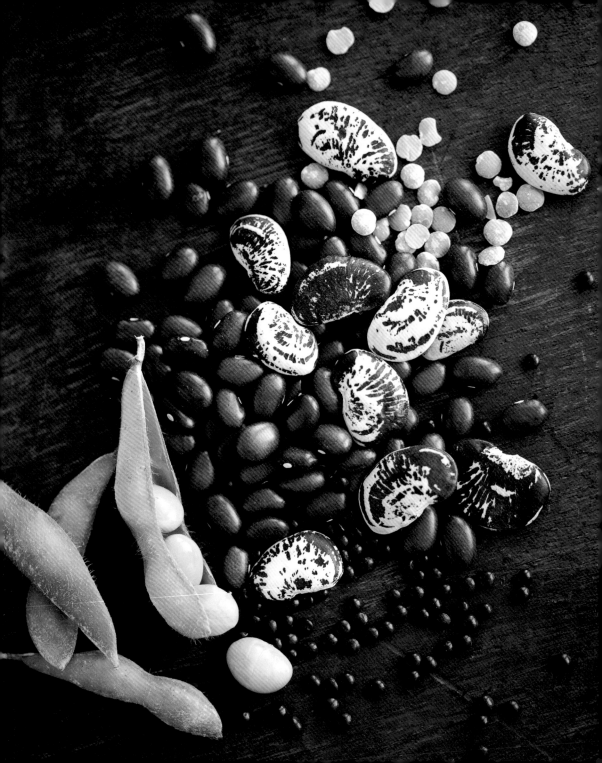

Soups

Basil-Spiked Tomato Soup

Quick and easy, this vibrant soup packs a super dose of tomatoes, a nutrition super food. For a fine meal, complement the dish with Honey-Glazed Green Beans with Almonds, page 147, and Roasted Garlic Bread, page 156. Note that you can puree the soup for a smoother texture if desired.

MAKES 4 SERVINGS

2 tablespoons extra-virgin olive oil
½ large yellow onion, finely diced
2 or 3 cloves garlic, minced
5 tablespoons finely chopped fresh
    basil, or 3 tablespoons dried basil
One 6-ounce can tomato paste
2 cups water

One 14.5-ounce can tomato sauce
One 14.5-ounce can diced low-
    sodium tomatoes
1 teaspoon salt
2 teaspoons freshly ground
    black pepper

> **♦ Nutrition Tip ♦**
>
> In Mediterranean countries where people eat a lot of tomatoes and other fruits and vegetables, cancer rates are lower.

- Heat the oil in a medium saucepan over medium heat. Sauté the onion and garlic for 3 to 5 minutes. Add the basil during the last minute of cooking time. Do not brown.

- Add the tomato paste. Cook for 1 minute.

- Add the water, tomato sauce, diced tomatoes, salt, and pepper. Cook until the soup simmers. Serve hot.

VARIATION

- Add reduced-fat milk or plain soy milk to the soup just before serving. Heat the milk before adding it and cook the soup, without boiling, for another 5 minutes.

PER SERVING (1 cup): 158 calories, 7 g fat, 5 g protein, 22 g carbohydrates, 6 g fiber, 1,473 mg sodium

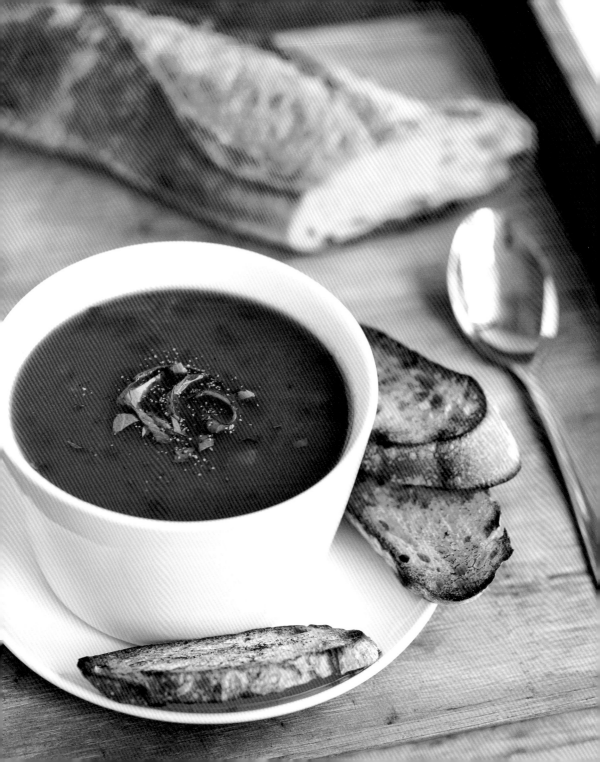

Masala Beet and Yogurt Soup

From Chef Jerry Traunfeld, Poppy Restaurant, and author of The Herbal Kitchen

Delight your senses with this unique blend of tastes. Pair the earthy, sweet taste of beets with classic Indian spices for a soup rich enough to be a meal.

MAKES 8 SERVINGS

4 green cardamom pods
2-inch cinnamon stick (preferably true cinnamon)
¼ star anise pod
1 tablespoon coriander seed
1½ teaspoons fennel seed
½ teaspoon cumin seed
½ teaspoon whole black peppercorns

3 tablespoons vegetable oil
1 large onion, peeled and chopped
4 cups peeled and cubed beets
1 tablespoon chopped fresh ginger
5 cups water
1½ teaspoons kosher salt
2 cups plain low-fat yogurt

• Place the cardamom pods, cinnamon stick, anise pod, coriander seed, fennel seed, cumin seed, and peppercorns in a small dry skillet over medium heat and shake until they are very fragrant and begin to turn a darker color. Transfer to a paper towel and cool. Put the spices in a rotary coffee grinder and grind until very fine.

• Heat the oil in a large saucepan over medium-high heat. Add the ground spices and onion and cook until the onion is softened and begins to brown. Add the beets, ginger, water, and salt. Bring to a boil, cover, and reduce the heat to low. Cook until the beets are very soft, about 30 minutes.

• Puree the soup in a blender in batches until very smooth. Return to the saucepan and whisk in the yogurt. Reheat the soup and serve hot. The soup can also be refrigerated and served chilled.

PER SERVING (1 cup): 137 calories, 7 g fat, 5 g protein, 16 g carbohydrates, 4 g fiber, 481 mg sodium

Black-Eyed Pea and Ham Soup

Any type of bean may be used in this easy one-pot meal, but black-eyed peas lend a distinctive flavor. Accompany the soup with a side of Quick Corn Bread, page 155.

MAKES 4 SERVINGS

8 cups water if using dried black-eyed peas, 2 cups if using canned beans
1 cup dried black-eyed peas, picked over and rinsed, or one 15-ounce can any type of beans
2 cups low-sodium, low-fat chicken stock or broth
¾ pound nitrate-free ham hock (optional)
1 onion, chopped

2 stalks celery, chopped
2 cloves garlic, minced
½ teaspoon freshly ground black pepper
1 bunch fresh kale, collard greens, or other green leafy vegetable, chopped
1 strip dried kombu seaweed (optional)

• If using dried black-eyed peas, bring 4 cups of the water to a boil and add the beans. Return to a boil, then remove the beans from the heat and drain. If using canned beans, omit this step and proceed with the recipe.

> ◆ Cooking Tip ◆
>
> Canned beans save a little time and taste almost as good as dried. If adding ham hock, be sure to remove the bone and skin after cooking.

• In a soup pot, combine the black-eyed peas with the remaining 4 cups water, or combine the canned beans with 2 cups water. Add the stock, ham hock, onion, celery, garlic, and pepper and bring to a boil. Reduce the heat and simmer for 1½ hours. Add the greens and kombu and cook for another 30 minutes, or until tender.

PER SERVING: 389 calories, 14 g fat, 30 g protein, 36 g carbohydrates, 7 g fiber, 287 mg sodium

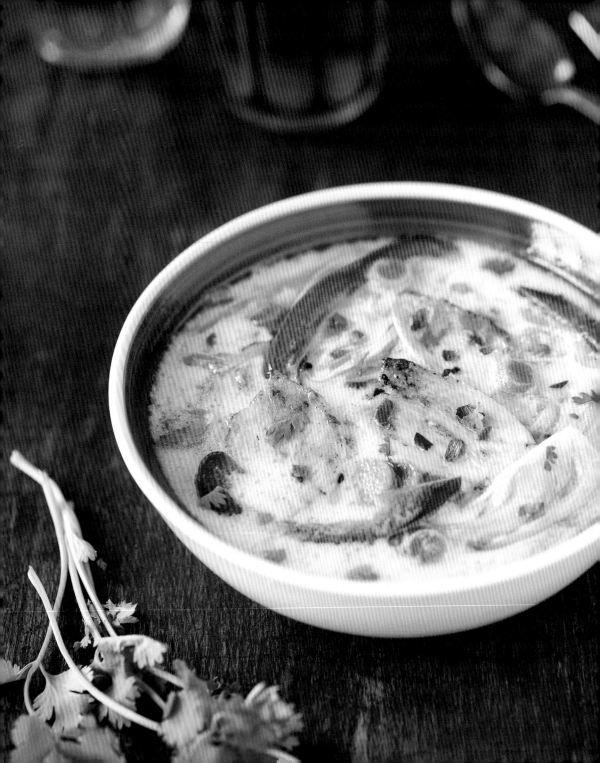

Thai Chicken Soup

From Chef Greg Atkinson, Restaurant Marché, and
  author of At the Kitchen Table

Coconut milk adds a subtle, creamy sweetness and the baby bok choy lends a tender crunch to this quick and savory soup.

MAKES 4 SERVINGS

4 cloves garlic
One 2-inch-long piece fresh ginger
2 tablespoons extra-virgin olive oil
1 small onion, peeled and thinly sliced
1 medium red bell pepper, seeded
  and sliced
1 medium carrot, peeled and sliced

One 6-ounce boneless chicken breast
  half, thinly sliced
15 ounces low-sodium chicken broth
  or stock
One 15-ounce can coconut milk
4 heads baby bok choy, sliced
A few leaves fresh cilantro
1 teaspoon crushed dried red chiles

• Rub the garlic and ginger through a very fine grater or put them in a blender with a couple tablespoons of water and puree until smooth.

• Heat the oil in a heavy-bottomed pot over medium-high heat and sauté the ginger and garlic for 1 minute, or until the aroma fills the air.

• Add the onion, bell pepper, and carrot to the pot and sauté for 1 minute longer. Add the chicken and cook for 5 minutes, turning the pieces 3 or 4 times as they begin to brown.

• Add the chicken broth and coconut milk and bring the soup to a boil. Add the baby bok choy and cook for 2 minutes, or until the bok choy is tender. Transfer the soup to serving bowls and top with cilantro leaves and crushed dried red chiles. Serve immediately.

PER SERVING: 268 calories, 10 g fat, 24 g protein, 28 g carbohydrates, 10 g fiber, 906 mg sodium

Shiitake Mushroom and Lentil Soup

From Margo Elbert, former Cancer Lifeline intern

The earthy and rustic flavors of this wholesome soup are so satisfying, you can serve the dish as a main course.

MAKES 6 SERVINGS

2 tablespoons extra-virgin olive oil
1 large red onion, finely chopped
4 cloves garlic, minced
1 large stalk celery, chopped
1 pound fresh shiitake mushrooms, stems removed and caps coarsely chopped
1 cup chopped canned tomatoes with their juices

1 cup dried brown lentils, picked over and rinsed
5 cups low-sodium vegetable stock or broth
Chopped hijiki or arame (optional)
Kosher or sea salt
½ cup chopped fresh parsley leaves

• Heat the oil in a heavy 4-quart saucepan over medium-high heat. Add the onion and garlic and cook, stirring, until they begin to soften, 2 to 3 minutes.

• Stir in the celery, and then add the mushrooms. Continue cooking, stirring occasionally, until the vegetables soften and begin to release their liquid, about 5 minutes.

• Stir in the tomatoes, lentils, and stock. For extra flavor, add the hijiki or arame. Bring to a boil.

• Reduce the heat to low, cover the pan, and simmer until the soup has thickened and the lentils are tender, about 1 hour. Add more stock if the soup is too thick.

• Season to taste with salt. Stir in the parsley and serve.

PER SERVING: 240 calories, 5 g fat, 10 g protein, 38 g carbohydrates, 13 g fiber, 200 mg sodium

"Cream" of Broccoli Soup

A delicious way to eat your green vegetables, this soup is easy to make, and any leftovers keep well in the refrigerator.

MAKES 6 SERVINGS

2 stems broccoli

4 cups low-sodium, nonfat chicken stock

2 tablespoons butter or no-trans-fat margarine

½ medium onion, chopped

2 tablespoons whole wheat pastry flour

2 cups nonfat milk

4 ounces part-skim mozzarella, grated

1 teaspoon salt (optional)

½ teaspoon curry powder

- Peel then chop the broccoli stems. Cook the broccoli in the chicken stock for about 20 minutes, or until tender. Strain the broccoli from the pan, reserving the liquid. Coarsely chop the broccoli and set aside.

- Melt the butter in a medium skillet over medium heat. Sauté the onion for about 5 minutes, or until transparent. Add the flour and stir until blended. Add the milk and continue stirring until heated through and the mixture thickens slightly.

- Remove from the heat and thoroughly blend in the cheese, salt to taste, and curry powder. Add the reserved cooking stock to the cheese mixture.

- Pour the soup in small batches into a food processor and blend slightly. Stir in the broccoli.

- If you need to reheat the soup before serving, be careful not to boil it.

PER SERVING (1 cup): 131 calories, 6 g fat, 11 g protein, 9 g carbohydrates, 2 g fiber, 586 mg sodium

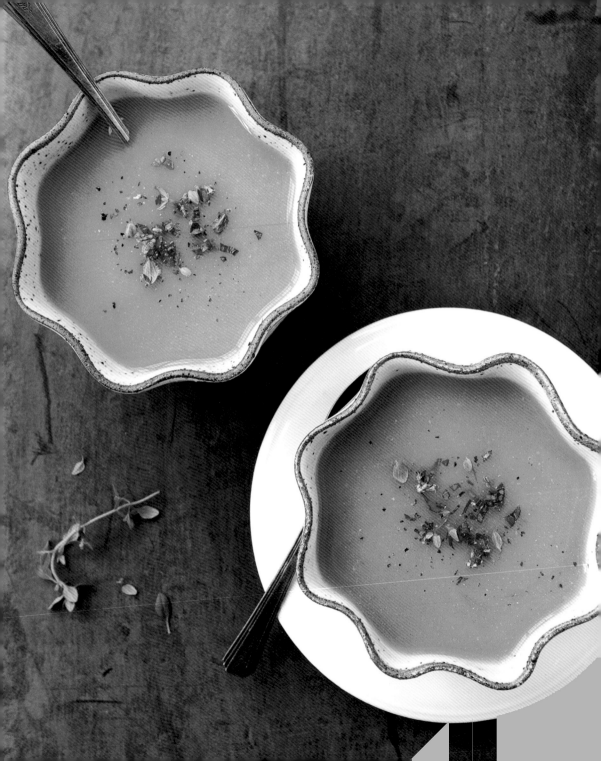

Golden Winter Squash Soup

Count on this colorful soup for a boost of important vitamins, minerals, and antioxidants.

MAKES 6 SERVINGS

2 teaspoons extra-virgin olive oil
1 large onion, finely chopped
2 carrots, peeled and finely chopped
2 stalks celery, trimmed and chopped
1 large sweet potato, peeled and cut
   into ½-inch cubes
1 butternut or hubbard squash,
   peeled, seeded, and cut into 1-inch
   cubes

Leaves from 4 sprigs fresh thyme, or
   1½ teaspoons dried thyme leaves
¼ teaspoon ground cloves
4 to 5 cups low-sodium vegetable
   broth
Salt and freshly ground black pepper
½ cup chopped fresh parsley leaves

- Heat the oil in a heavy 4-quart saucepan over medium-high heat. Add the onion, carrots, celery, and sweet potato and cook, stirring, until they begin to soften, 3 to 4 minutes.

- Add the squash, thyme, cloves, and broth, and season to taste with salt.

- Increase the heat to high and bring to a boil. Reduce the heat to medium-low, partially cover the pan, and simmer until the squash is tender when pierced with a sharp knife tip, about 20 minutes.

> **♦ Cooking Tip ♦**
>
> To save energy, cut the squash in half, seed, and place in a baking dish, flesh side down. Add water to cover the bottom of the dish. Cover the dish and bake in a 350-degree-F oven for 25 to 30 minutes, or until the squash is soft. Scoop out the flesh and add to the saucepan with the sweet potato in the first step.

- Transfer the soup to a food processor or blender, or use an immersion blender, and process to the desired consistency.

- Return the soup to the pan and season to taste with pepper.

- Stir in the chopped parsley. Reheat before serving.

PER SERVING: 150 calories, 2 g fat, 4 g protein, 29 g carbohydrates, 4 g fiber, 100 mg sodium

Black Bean Soup

This tasty soup is packed with four of our Top 10 "Super Foods": garlic, a cruciferous vegetable (kale), mushrooms, and black beans. The bonus is that preparation takes only about half an hour.

MAKES 8 SERVINGS

½ medium onion, chopped (about 1 cup)
2 cloves garlic, chopped
2 stalks celery, chopped
½ bunch organic kale (stems removed) or 3 to 4 ounces bok choy, finely chopped
1 cup fresh shiitake or button mushrooms, stemmed and cut into small pieces
½ teaspoon ground cumin
4 cups low-sodium chicken stock or vegetable stock, divided
Two 15-ounce cans low-sodium black beans
1 cup water
Plain low-fat yogurt
Chopped parsley

- In a large nonstick skillet, cook the onion, garlic, celery, kale, mushrooms, and cumin in 2 tablespoons of the chicken stock for about 10 minutes, or until soft.

- Add the remaining stock, beans, and water. Simmer for 20 minutes.

- Transfer the soup to serving bowls and top with a dollop of yogurt and a sprinkle of parsley.

PER SERVING (1 cup): 96 calories, 1 g fat, 8 g protein, 19 g carbohydrates, 6 g fiber, 275 mg sodium

Tofu Miso Soup

A simple soup that combines the nutritious properties of tofu and sea vegetables with the rich flavor of miso.

MAKES 4 SERVINGS

3-inch strip dried kombu or wakame seaweed
3½ cups water, divided
½ cup grated carrot
½ cup chopped bok choy or kale

¼ cup thinly sliced green onion (green and white parts)
½ cup cubed reduced-fat, firm silken tofu
1 tablespoon brown miso

- Soak the dried seaweed in ½ cup water for 5 minutes. Drain and cut the seaweed into small pieces with scissors.

- In a large pot over medium heat, bring the remaining 3 cups water to a boil. Add the seaweed and carrot and simmer for 5 minutes.

- Stir in the bok choy and cook for 5 minutes. Add the green onion and tofu and simmer for 5 minutes.

- Remove from the heat and gently dissolve the miso into the soup. If you need to reheat the soup before serving, take care not to let it boil.

PER SERVING: 43 calories, 2 g fat, 3 g protein, 4 g carbohydrates, 1 g fiber, 186 mg sodium

♦ Nutrition Tip ♦

Miso is a paste made from grains and fermented soybeans. It comes in red, brown, or yellow varieties, depending upon the type of grain that has been added to the soybeans. This recipe calls for brown miso, which is made with barley.

Chilled Avocado Soup

Rich, creamy, and lightly spiced, this soup makes a meal when paired with a generous salad of mixed organic greens.

MAKES 4 SERVINGS

2 ripe avocados, peeled and pitted
1 cup soy milk or reduced-fat milk
¼ cup cilantro leaves
1 tablespoon finely minced fresh
   ginger
Juice from 1 lemon (about
   2 tablespoons)

½ teaspoon Asian chili sauce
1 teaspoon salt
½ cup plain low-fat Greek yogurt
2 cups vegetable stock or low-
   sodium, nonfat chicken stock
½ cup finely chopped red bell pepper,
   for garnish

- Put the avocados in a food processor and puree until smooth. Add the soy milk, cilantro, ginger, lemon juice, chili sauce, and salt. Process until smooth.

- With the machine running, pour the yogurt and stock through the feed tube.

- Transfer to a resealable container and refrigerate until thoroughly chilled.

- Transfer the soup into serving bowls and place a little chopped bell pepper in the center. Serve immediately.

PER SERVING: 230 calories, 17 g fat, 7 g protein, 15 g carbohydrates, 7 g fiber, 720 mg sodium

> ◆ **Nutrition Tip** ◆
>
> Greek yogurt is higher in protein
> than most other yogurts.

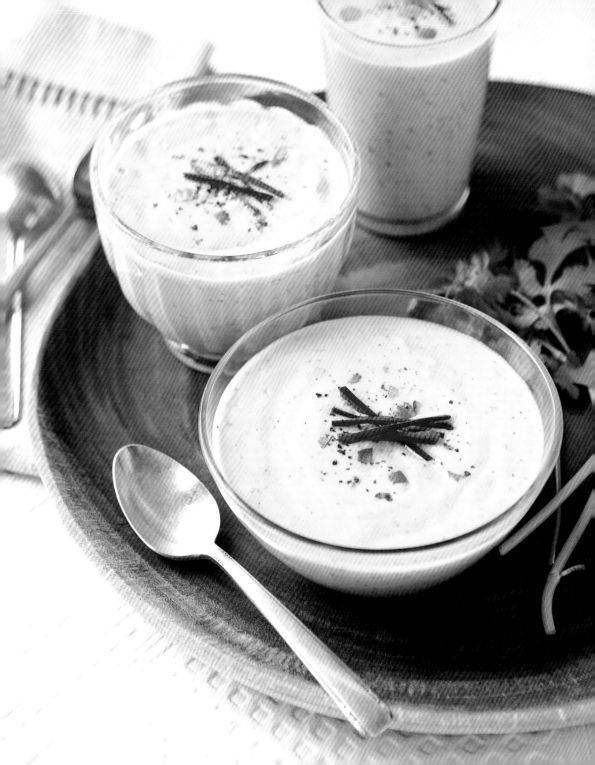

Gingered Carrot Soup

This is a fast and easy soup. Preparation takes 5 minutes and cooking time is just 15 to 20 minutes. Plus the delicate play between the spice of the ginger and the sweetness of the carrots makes this soup a menu choice for all seasons. Serve it cold in the spring and summer and warm in the fall and winter

MAKES 6 SERVINGS

2 tablespoons extra-virgin olive oil, divided
1 small onion, chopped
2 cloves garlic, crushed
1 pound (about 6 medium) carrots, peeled and sliced

2 teaspoons minced or grated fresh ginger
4 cups low-sodium chicken broth or stock
2 cups plain soy milk or nonfat milk
Salt and freshly ground black pepper

> **• Nutrition Tip •**
>
> Like other deep orange vegetables, carrots contain antioxidants. Many studies have reported a relation-ship between low risk for cancer and high consump-tion of foods containing antioxidants.

- Heat 1 tablespoon of the oil in a large stockpot over medium heat. Add the onion and garlic and cook until they are soft.

- Add the carrots, ginger, and chicken broth to the pot. Simmer until the carrots are tender, about 10 minutes.

- Pulse the soup in a food processor or blender. Add the soy milk, remaining 1 tablespoon oil, and salt and pepper to taste and blend until the soup is smooth. Serve hot, or chill and serve cold.

PER SERVING (1 cup): 140 calories, 9 g fat, 5 g protein, 12 g carbohydrates, 3 g fiber, 140 mg sodium

Vegetables and Sides

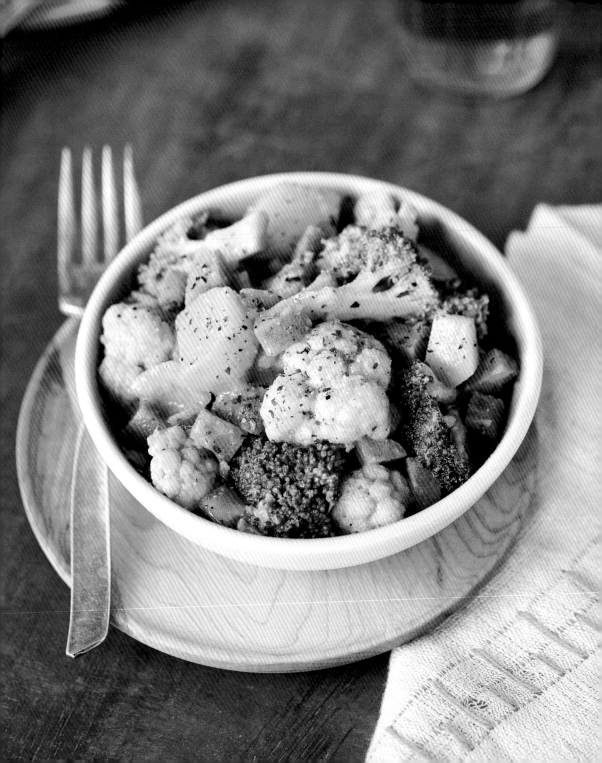

Curried Root Vegetables

From Ami Karnosh, CN, Cancer Lifeline Nutrition Educator

Curries come in hundreds of varieties, in both powder and paste form. Pick your curry of choice—hot, spicy, or mild—and pair it up with coconut milk for a smooth, mellow flavor. Explore the world of curries with this flavorful vegetable dish.

MAKES 4 SERVINGS

1 tablespoon vegetable oil or ghee (clarified butter)
1 medium onion, diced (about 1 cup)
1 large skin-on potato, diced (about 1 cup)
1 large carrot, diced (about 1 cup)
1 parsnip, turnip, or rutabaga, diced (about 1 cup)

Optional vegetables: 1 cup diced winter squash, beets, cauliflower, broccoli, peas, or mushrooms
1½ tablespoons curry powder
1 teaspoon ground cumin
1 cup or more coconut milk
2 teaspoons tamari or low-sodium soy sauce
Freshly ground black pepper

• In a large saucepan, heat the oil over medium heat. Add the onion, potato, carrot, parsnip, and any additional vegetables. Stir in the curry powder and cumin. Stir in the coconut milk, cover, and let simmer for about 20 minutes, or until the potato can be easily pierced with a fork.

• Thin the sauce with water, if desired. Season with the tamari, pepper, and any other seasonings to taste.

PER SERVING (½ cup): 290 calories, 16 g fat, 5 g protein, 34 g carbohydrates, 6 g fiber, 210 mg sodium

♦ Nutrition Note ♦

Ghee is clarified butter; the milk solids and water are boiled off, leaving just the butterfat. This dish is suitable for people who are on casein-free diets.

Oven-Roasted Vegetables

From Marianne Sakamoto, cancer survivor

Roasting vegetables heightens their flavor and works well for many types. Vary the recipe according to the season. In winter, try root vegetables such as turnips and yams. In summer, add plum tomatoes, and in spring, add cremini mushrooms.

MAKES 8 SERVINGS

1 medium green bell pepper, seeded and cut into strips
1 medium red bell pepper, seeded and cut into strips
1 medium yellow bell pepper, seeded and cut into strips
3 small potatoes, quartered
2 medium carrots, peeled, halved lengthwise, and quartered
1 large onion, quartered
2 or 3 cloves garlic, chopped
2 to 3 tablespoons extra-virgin olive oil
¼ teaspoon each of assorted dried herbs: basil, oregano, thyme, rosemary
Kosher or sea salt and freshly ground black pepper

- Preheat the oven to 350 degrees F.

- Put all the vegetables in a large resealable plastic bag and add the oil, herbs, and salt and pepper to taste. Seal the bag and shake to coat the vegetables.

- Spread the vegetables on a rimmed baking sheet.

- Bake, stirring every 20 minutes, until the vegetables are browned at the edges and soft.

PER SERVING: 113 calories, 5 g fat, 2 g protein, 15 g carbohydrates, 3 g fiber, 11 mg sodium

♦ Contributor Tip ♦

The vegetables can be eaten as is or added to soups, stews, or pasta. It's an easy recipe—and no mess.

Indian-Style Roasted Cauliflower

From Ami Karnosh, CN, Cancer Lifeline Nutrition Educator

Cauliflower is one of the "super foods" of the broccoli family. Serve this colorful Indian-spiced dish with Creamy Polenta and Bean Casserole, page 197, for a satisfying meal.

MAKES 4 SERVINGS

1 small head cauliflower, cut into large pieces (about 2 cups)
2 tablespoons grapeseed, coconut, or canola oil, or ¼ cup water or broth

2 teaspoons curry powder
2 teaspoons garam masala
1 teaspoon ground turmeric
½ teaspoon sea salt

- Preheat the oven to 425 degrees F.

- In a large baking dish, combine all the ingredients and toss until the cauliflower is well coated.

- Bake for 10 minutes and then stir. Bake for another 10 minutes, or until the cauliflower is fork-tender.

PER SERVING (½ cup): 80 calories, 7 g fat, 1 g protein, 4 g carbohydrates, 1 g fiber, 310 mg sodium

Alternatively, you can cook this on the stovetop: Heat the grapeseed oil in a large pan over medium-high heat. Add the cauliflower and spices and cook for about 15 minutes, or until the cauliflower is fork-tender.

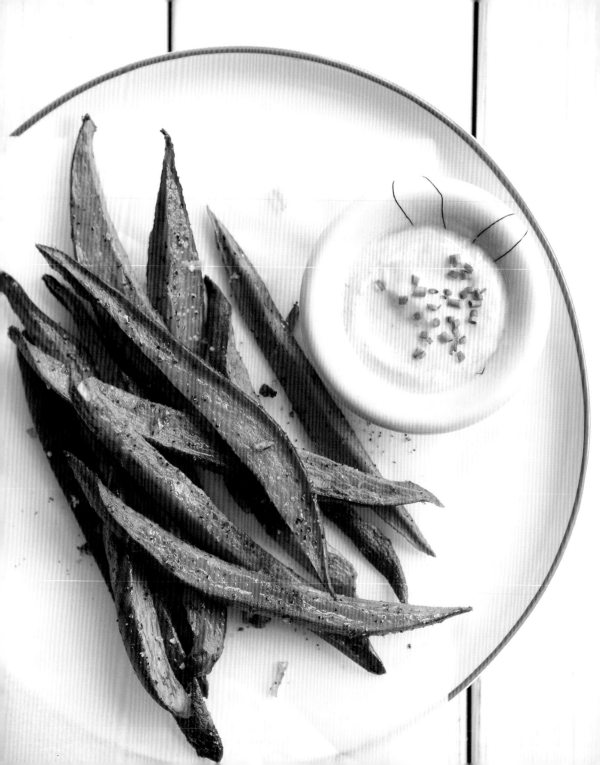

Baked Sweet Potato Fries

Enjoy these oven-baked sweet potatoes, packed with high-grade nutrition and A+ taste. White potatoes may also be used here, or try a combination of white and sweet potatoes.

MAKES 4 SERVINGS

2 medium organic sweet potatoes or yams, well scrubbed (and peeled if non-organic)
2 teaspoons extra-virgin olive oil
2 teaspoons dried minced onion

½ teaspoon salt
½ teaspoon freshly ground black pepper
½ teaspoon garlic powder

• Preheat the oven to 375 degrees F. Line a rimmed baking sheet with parchment paper or spray with nonstick cooking spray.

• Slice each potato in half, then slice each half lengthwise into 4 or 5 pieces. They should resemble steak fries.

• Place the potatoes in a bowl and coat well with the oil.

• In another small bowl, mix together the dried minced onion, salt, pepper, and garlic powder. Sprinkle over the potatoes and toss well, making sure to distribute the seasonings evenly.

• Arrange the potatoes on the baking sheet and bake, stirring once or twice, for 20 to 30 minutes. Serve immediately.

PER SERVING: 80 calories, 2 g fat, 2 g protein, 14 g carbohydrates, 2 g fiber, 310 mg sodium

Arame-Stuffed Mushroom Caps

From the company chefs at Eden Foods

Arame is a mild-tasting sea vegetable that is pre-toasted, so it cooks quickly. Pair the rich, meaty texture of this mushroom dish with a soup, such as Gingered Carrot Soup, page 136.

MAKES 6 SERVINGS

1 cup arame, rinsed, soaked in cold water for 5 minutes, then drained

2 cups water

18 large white button or cremini mushrooms (about 2½-inch diameter)

1 teaspoon light sesame oil

1 medium onion, minced

¼ cup mirin

Juice from 1 lemon (about 3 tablespoons)

2 teaspoons low-sodium soy sauce

Juice from 1 teaspoon grated fresh ginger (use a garlic press to squeeze out the juice; discard the pulp)

¼ cup chopped fresh parsley, for garnish

- Preheat the oven to 350 degrees F.

- Place the arame and water in a saucepan. Cover and cook over medium heat for 15 minutes. Rinse, drain, and mince the arame.

- Stem the mushrooms and place the caps in a 2-quart baking dish. Chop the stems.

- Heat the oil in a skillet and sauté the onion and mushroom stems for 3 to 5 minutes. Be careful not to overcook. Add the arame.

- In a small bowl, combine the mirin, lemon juice, soy sauce, and ginger juice. Pour half of this marinade over the arame, stir, and cook until the liquid evaporates.

- Stuff the mushroom caps with the arame mixture. Pour a little of the remaining marinade over each mushroom cap.

- Bake for 20 to 25 minutes. Garnish the mushrooms with the parsley and serve.

PER SERVING: 71 calories, 1 g fat, 4 g protein, 15 g carbohydrates, 4 g fiber, 256 mg sodium

Ruby Chard with Garlic, Chile, and Lemon

*From Chef Tom Douglas, James Beard award winner and owner
of ten Seattle restaurants*

A brilliant vegetable, chard comes in a variety of hues, including red, yellow, and green. Serve this lovely dish with Herb-Roasted Chicken, page 170.

MAKES 4 SERVINGS

3 bunches (about 2 pounds) ruby or other chard, washed, stemmed, and roughly chopped (about 12 cups loosely packed)
¼ cup extra-virgin olive oil
¼ teaspoon crushed red pepper flakes
2 teaspoons minced garlic
Kosher salt and freshly ground black pepper
1 lemon, quartered

- Pat the chopped chard leaves with paper towels to soak up excess moisture.

- Heat the oil and red pepper flakes in a large sauté pan over medium-high heat, stirring occasionally, for 3 to 5 minutes.

- Add the chard (in batches as needed) and garlic to the pan and cook, stirring frequently, for 3 to 5 minutes. When the leaves are wilted, season to taste with salt and pepper, squeeze the lemon wedges over the top, and toss well.

- Divide the chard among 4 plates and serve immediately.

> **♦ Chef's Tip ♦**
>
> Use a large, deep pan for cooking the chard, or cook it in batches. To make chard for more than four people, blanch it first in a pot of boiling water, shock it in ice water, squeeze all the water out, and pat dry with paper towels. Reheat the chard by sautéing it in olive oil and garlic.

PER SERVING: 174 calories, 15 g fat, 4 g protein, 10 g carbohydrates, 4 g fiber, 484 mg sodium

Garlic-Sautéed Greens

Discover the exciting flavor of leafy greens. Mix and match a variety of seasonal greens for this quick sauté.

MAKES 4 SERVINGS

1 tablespoon extra-virgin olive oil
8 cups sliced raw greens, such as kale, chard, collards, mustard greens, and broccoli rabe (1½-inch slices)

3 green onions (green and white parts), chopped (about ½ cup)
2 large cloves garlic, chopped
Salt and freshly ground black pepper

- Heat the oil in a large, heavy skillet over medium-high heat. Add the greens and green onions and cook, stirring frequently, for 2 minutes, or until all the greens are heated.

- Add the garlic and stir. When the greens have turned bright green and begun to wilt, season to taste with salt and pepper. Sauté a few minutes longer. Serve immediately.

PER SERVING: 107 calories, 4 g fat, 5 g protein, 15 g carbohydrates, 3 g fiber, 61 mg sodium

Phytochemicals called indoles give leafy greens such as kale, collards, mustard greens, and broccoli their "bite."

Honey-Glazed Green Beans with Almonds

Crisp, slightly sweet green beans with a crunch of almonds make this recipe a winner.

MAKES 4 SERVINGS

2 cups fresh or frozen green beans
1 tablespoon butter or no-trans-fat margarine
1 medium shallot, minced

2 tablespoons water
1 tablespoon honey or sugar
¼ cup sliced almonds

- Place the beans in a steamer basket over boiling water and steam until tender, about 3 to 5 minutes.

- Melt the butter in a medium skillet over medium heat. Add the shallot and cook for 5 minutes, or until translucent.

- Add the water, honey, and almonds and cook for 2 minutes.

- Add the steamed beans to the pan and stir until coated. Serve hot.

PER SERVING (½ cup): 100 calories, 6 g fat, 3 g protein, 12 g carbohydrates, 3 g fiber, 30 mg sodium

Broccoli with Sesame-Crusted Tofu

Tofu takes on a medley of flavors from a sesame-ginger marinade, and broccoli offers a generous serving of health-boosting green vegetables.

MAKES 4 SERVINGS

3 cloves garlic, minced
½ cup balsamic vinegar
¼ cup low-sodium soy sauce
1 tablespoon toasted sesame oil
1 tablespoon grated fresh ginger

1 pound firm tofu, cut into ½-inch pieces
4 heads broccoli
1 red onion, sliced
1 red or yellow bell pepper, sliced thin
½ teaspoon sesame seeds

- To marinate the tofu, mix the garlic, balsamic vinegar, soy sauce, oil, and grated ginger in a shallow bowl. Add the tofu and stir well to coat. Cover and refrigerate for at least 30 minutes. If you prefer to serve this dish hot, heat the tofu in the microwave for 2 minutes.

- To prepare the broccoli, trim and peel the stems and cut the broccoli into 2-inch pieces.

- Steam the broccoli florets and stems in a steamer basket over boiling water until slightly crunchy, about 5 minutes. Let cool.

♦ Cooking Tip ♦

Make this a super-quick recipe by using packaged baked tofu instead of marinating it yourself. It can be found in a variety of flavors.

- In a medium bowl, toss the onion and bell pepper with the broccoli.

- Using a slotted spoon, remove the tofu from the marinade and add to the broccoli. Sprinkle with the sesame seeds and serve.

PER SERVING: 217 calories, 10 g fat, 15 g protein, 23 g carbohydrates, 7 g fiber, 658 mg sodium

Grilled and Roasted Walla Walla Sweet Onions with Pine Nut Butter

From Chef Tom Douglas, James Beard award winner and owner
of ten Seattle restaurants

Walla Walla onions are featured in this recipe, but you can substitute Vidalia, Maui, or Bermuda onions. Present the roasted onions on a bed of Ruby Chard with Garlic, Chile, and Lemon, page 145, or serve on Polenta Squares, page 161.

MAKES 4 SERVINGS

½ cup (about 2½ ounces) pine nuts, toasted

3 tablespoons unsalted butter, at room temperature

1 teaspoon grated lemon zest

½ teaspoon chopped fresh rosemary

¼ teaspoon freshly ground black pepper

¼ teaspoon kosher salt

4 Walla Walla onions

Extra-virgin olive oil

- To make the pine nut butter, chop half of the pine nuts. In a small bowl, use a wooden spoon to mix together the whole and chopped pine nuts, butter, lemon zest, rosemary, pepper, and salt. Set aside.

- To prepare the onions, preheat the grill to high heat and preheat the oven to 400 degrees F.

- Peel the onions and cut them in half lengthwise. Leave the root ends intact so the onions hold together. Brush the onion halves with oil and grill, cut side down, until lightly marked, about 3 minutes.

- Transfer the onion halves, cut side up, to a baking sheet, place in the oven, and roast until soft and cooked through, 30 to 40 minutes.

- Alternatively, instead of grilling them, you can sear the onions in 2 tablespoons oil in an ovenproof frying pan over medium-high heat. Sear the cut

continued

sides until brown, about 3 minutes. Flip the onions and place in the oven to roast as directed.

• Remove the onions from the oven. Spread the cut halves liberally with the nut butter. Return to the oven to melt and bake in the butter, about 5 minutes.

PER SERVING: 260 calories, 21 g fat, 6 g protein, 16 g carbohydrates, 4 g fiber, 124 mg sodium

◆ Chef's Tip ◆

The nut butter can be made a few days ahead and stored, tightly wrapped, in the refrigerator or in the freezer for a few weeks. The onions can be grilled and roasted a few hours ahead and kept at room temperature. Return them to the oven to warm them through before spreading with the nut butter.

Roasted Beets and Beet Greens with Marcona Almonds and Zolfini Beans

From Chef Holly Smith, Cafe Juanita, Seattle

Warm, rich colors and flavors are combined in this winning recipe.

MAKES 4 SERVINGS

3 bunches baby beets with greens
(if the tops are skimpy, add chopped
kale, ruby chard, or turnip greens)

¼ cup extra-virgin olive oil, plus more
for dressing sliced beet

2 cloves garlic, minced

2 shallots, minced

¾ cup cooked zolfini beans (see
Chef's Note)

2 teaspoons chopped fresh marjoram

Kosher salt and freshly ground black
pepper

Juice from ½ lemon (about
1 tablespoon)

1 large red beet, roasted, peeled, and
sliced ⅛ to ¼ inch thick (at room
temperature for serving)

½ cup Marcona almonds, toasted

- Preheat the oven to 400 degrees F.

- Remove the baby beets from their greens. Stem and wash the greens.

- Wash the beets and place in a roasting pan. Cover the beets halfway with water. Cover the pan with foil and roast the beets in the oven until tender, 20 to 30 minutes.

- Remove the outer skin from the warm beets. (Be aware that they stain, so wear gloves if possible and peel the beets on a wipeable surface.) Cut the beets into halves or quarters, depending on their size.

- Heat the oil in a large sauté pan over medium heat. Add the garlic and shallots. Let them sweat in the oil for 3 minutes, or until the garlic begins to turn slightly golden.

continued

- Add the beet greens and zolfini beans to the pan. Add the marjoram, salt to taste, and the roasted baby beets. Toss well and warm through. Season to taste with additional salt, pepper, and lemon juice.

- Turn off the heat and keep the mixture warm in the pan.

- Dress the room-temperature beet slices with a little extra-virgin olive oil and a pinch of salt and pepper.

- Place a beet slice on each of 4 plates. Top each slice with some of the warm beet mixture. Garnish with the Marcona almonds and, if desired, a final drizzle of best-quality extra-virgin olive oil.

PER SERVING: 410 calories, 24 g fat, 15 g protein, 41 g carbohydrates, 15 g fiber, 629 mg sodium

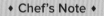

♦ Chef's Note ♦

Zolfini beans are grown in Tuscany. You may substitute cooked white beans, kidney beans, or garbanzos for the zolfini beans. Marcona almonds, grown in Spain, are considered to have more flavor due to higher fat content. Other varieties of almonds can be used instead.

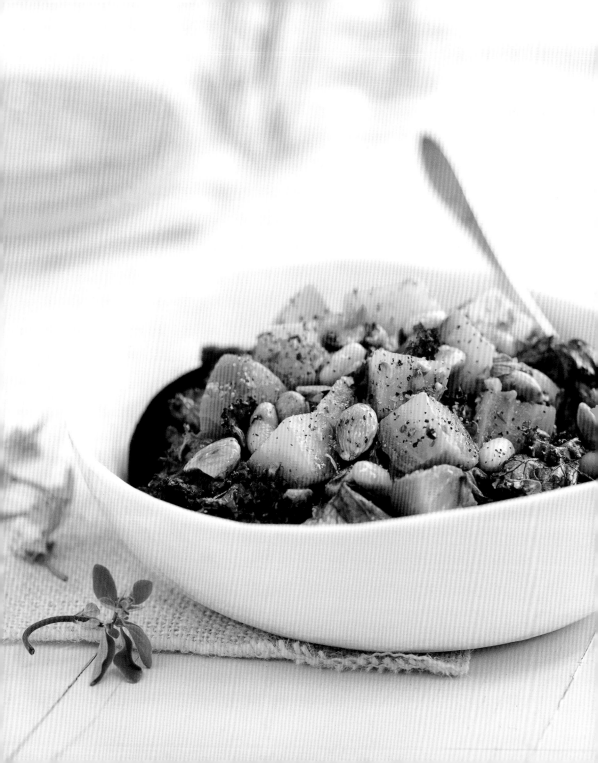

Stuffed Baked Potatoes with Nori

From Margo Elbert, former Cancer Lifeline intern

Baked potatoes take on a delectable new flavor with the addition of a sea vegetable. Nori is one of the richest sea-vegetable sources of protein.

MAKES 6 SERVINGS

6 medium potatoes
6 pearl onions
1 bulb garlic, top sliced off and
    unpeeled cloves separated
¼ cup white miso

¼ cup cold-pressed extra-virgin
    olive oil
1 cup roasted nori, flaked or cut into
    strips (see Cooking Tip), divided

> ♦ **Cooking Tip** ♦
>
> To cut the nori, stack several sheets of nori (a standard sheet is 7 by 8 inches) and cut them all at once. With the short side toward you, use scissors to cut into 8 equal strips about 1 inch wide. Stack the strips and cut them into ½-inch lengths to make ½-inch-by-1-inch pieces.

- Preheat the oven to 350 degrees F.

- Lightly oil a pie pan or roasting pan. Place the potatoes, onions, and garlic cloves in the pan.

- Roast for 45 minutes, or until tender. Set aside until cool enough to handle.

- Cut each potato in half lengthwise and scoop the flesh into a large mixing bowl, reserving the emptied skins. Remove the outer onion skins and cut the onions into small pieces, adding them to the bowl. Squeeze the garlic cloves from their skins and add to the bowl.

- In a small bowl, whisk together the miso and oil.

- Stir the miso mixture and ½ cup of the roasted nori into the potato mixture. Mash together until well blended.

- Spoon the filling into the potato skins, making slight mounds. Garnish with the remaining ½ cup roasted nori and serve.

PER SERVING: 334 calories, 10 g fat, 7 g protein, 56 g carbohydrates, 6 g fiber, 337 mg sodium

Quick Corn Bread

From Margo Elbert, former Cancer Lifeline intern

The title says it all: this corn bread is quick and easy to make. Serve as an accompaniment to Grilled and Roasted Walla Walla Sweet Onions with Pine Nut Butter, page 149, or Three-Bean Vegetarian Chili, page 205.

MAKES 8 SERVINGS

1 cup fresh or thawed frozen corn
¾ cup finely ground cornmeal
¾ cup whole wheat flour
¼ cup unbleached all-purpose flour or soy flour
¼ cup polenta

1 tablespoon baking powder
½ teaspoon baking soda
½ teaspoon salt
1 cup plain soy milk
2 tablespoons honey
2 tablespoons canola oil

- Preheat the oven to 350 degrees F. Lightly oil a 9-by-5-inch or 11-by-3-inch loaf pan.

- Put the corn in a small bowl and allow it to sit and collect juices.

- In a large mixing bowl, whisk together the cornmeal, whole wheat and all-purpose flours, polenta, baking powder, baking soda, and salt.

- In a medium bowl, beat together the soy milk, honey, oil, and 2 tablespoons liquid drained from the corn (add water as needed to supplement).

- Add the wet ingredients to the cornmeal mixture, stirring just until moist, and then fold in the corn kernels.

- Using a spatula, scrape the batter into the prepared pan and bake until a knife inserted in the center comes out clean, 35 to 40 minutes. Let cool on a rack.

- When completely cool, turn the corn bread out onto a cutting board or platter. Cut into 8 slices and serve.

PER SERVING (1 slice): 193 calories, 5 g fat, 5 g protein, 33 g carbohydrates, 4 g fiber, 468 mg sodium

Roasted Garlic Bread

A crusty whole grain bread infused with olive oil and garlic, this is the perfect accompaniment for any salad. Try pairing it with Spinach Salad with Poppy Seed Balsamic Vinaigrette, page 106. The roasted garlic can be made ahead of time and stored, drizzled with olive oil, in an airtight container in the refrigerator for up to one week.

MAKES 7 SERVINGS

¼ cup extra-virgin olive oil
¼ cup Worcestershire sauce
2 tablespoons low-sodium soy sauce
   or Bragg Liquid Aminos
2 tablespoons water

1 teaspoon dried dill
Roasted Garlic (recipe follows)
1 whole wheat sourdough baguette
   (about 14 ounces), sliced lengthwise

• Preheat the oven to 350 degrees F.

• Combine the oil, Worcestershire, soy sauce, water, and dill in a small saucepan over medium heat. Squeeze the roasted cloves into the pan, mash, and stir until heated through.

• Spread the garlic mixture evenly over both halves of the baguette.

• Fit the loaf back together and slice it crosswise into 1-inch-thick slices. Wrap the whole loaf in foil and bake for about 30 minutes.

PER SERVING: 220 calories, 12 g fat, 4 g protein, 24 g carbohydrates, 1 g fiber, 480 mg sodium

ROASTED GARLIC

3 bulbs garlic, tops sliced off

About 2 tablespoons extra-virgin olive oil

• Preheat the oven to 350 degrees F. Place the garlic bulbs root end down in a small baking dish. Drizzle with just enough oil to seep into the sleeves, and roast until the cloves are bubbling brown and bulging, about 40 minutes. Let cool.

Cooking Whole Grains: Brown Rice, Millet, Quinoa, and Buckwheat

WHOLE GRAINS CONTAIN A RICH VARIETY OF VITAMINS, MINERALS, phytochemicals, and fiber. Processed grains like white flour or white rice lack the nutritional value of whole grains. Onion, garlic, or other chopped vegetables may be added to the grains before cooking. Seaweed, an excellent source of calcium, can also be added. (For dishes that cook longer than an hour, just cut the seaweed into small pieces and toss it in. For dishes that cook for less than an hour, soak the seaweed for 10 minutes, or until it is soft enough to cut, then cut it up and throw it in.) For consistent quality, consider using a rice cooker. Make a large batch of your favorite grains and freeze in one- or two-serving containers for quick meal preparation. Thaw in the microwave or heat on the stovetop.

Brown Rice

2 cups water, or 1 cup low-sodium, nonfat chicken stock and 1 cup water

Pinch of sea salt

1 cup short- or long-grain brown rice

For larger batches, use less water proportionately. For example:

5½ cups water, or 2 cups low-sodium, nonfat chicken stock and 3½ cups water

⅛ teaspoon sea salt

3 cups short- or long-grain brown rice

- Rinse the rice and let drain in a strainer.

- Bring the water and salt to a boil in a medium saucepan over medium heat. Add the rice and cover. Reduce the heat to medium-low and simmer undisturbed for 50 to 60 minutes.

PER SERVING (½ cup): 110 calories, 1 g fat, 2 g protein, 24 g carbohydrates, 1 g fiber, 50 mg sodium

◆ Nutrition Tip ◆

For more flavor and extra fiber, minerals, and protein, try adding other grains to plain boiled rice. Rye or wheat berries, dried corn, sweet brown rice, barley, lentils, kombu seaweed pieces, and wild rice all work well. Simply presoak ¼ cup of any selected grain for several hours, or bring the grain to a boil in a covered pan, simmer for 5 minutes, and set aside for 1 hour. Drain and then add the grain to 1 cup of uncooked rice and boil as instructed.

Millet

MAKES 8 SERVINGS

3 cups water   1 cup millet
Pinch of sea salt

• Bring the water and salt to a boil in a medium saucepan over medium heat.
  Add the millet and cover. Reduce the heat to medium-low and simmer for
  25 minutes.

PER SERVING (½ cup): 90 calories, 1 g fat, 3 g protein,
18 g carbohydrates, 2 g fiber, 40 mg sodium

> **• Cooking Tip •**
>
> For a fluffier millet, dry-roast the grain in a skil-
> let over medium heat, stirring it until it smells
> toasty. Proceed with the recipe as instructed.

Quinoa

The name of this ancient grain is pronounced "keen-wah."

MAKES 8 SERVINGS

2¼ cups water   1 cup quinoa
Pinch of sea salt

• Bring the water and salt to a boil in a medium saucepan over medium heat.
  Add the quinoa and cover. Reduce the heat to medium-low and simmer for
  20 minutes.

PER SERVING (½ cup): 156 calories, 2.5 g fat, 6 g protein,
27 g carbohydrates, 3 g fiber, 2 mg sodium

Buckwheat

MAKES 2 TO 3 SERVINGS

1 cup raw buckwheat groats
2 cups water

Pinch of sea salt

- Dry-roast the buckwheat in a medium skillet over medium heat, stirring until brown.
- Bring the water and salt to a boil in a medium saucepan over medium heat. Add the buckwheat and cover. Reduce the heat to medium-low and simmer for 20 minutes.

PER SERVING: 292 calories, 3 g fat, 11 g protein, 61 g carbohydrates, 9 g fiber, 8 mg sodium

Polenta Squares

Polenta can be a quick and satisfying meal when combined with cheese and served with vegetables, beans, or a salad. If refrigerated, polenta keeps for three to five days. To reheat, pop in the microwave for about thirty seconds. Top with your favorite tomato sauce.

MAKES 4 SERVINGS

2 cups low-sodium chicken
   stock or broth
1½ cups water
1¼ cups polenta

Optional Additions
¼ cup grated part-skim mozzarella,
   ricotta, or Parmesan cheese
1 fresh tomato, sliced
1 clove garlic, minced
½ teaspoon chopped fresh basil

- Put the stock and water in a medium saucepan over medium heat. Add the polenta and bring to a boil, whisking constantly.

- Cook, stirring frequently, for about 5 minutes, or until thick and smooth.

- Stir in any optional ingredients and remove the pan from the heat.

- Spread the mixture in a lightly oiled 8-inch square baking dish. Let stand for 20 minutes, or until firm. Cut into squares.

PER SERVING (4-by-4 square): 205 calories, 3 g fat, 8 g protein, 36 g carbohydrates, 4 g fiber, 80 mg sodium

♦ Cooking Tip ♦

This corn porridge can be made on the stovetop in less than fifteen minutes. The consistency may vary from dense and firm to soft and creamy. The texture softens with longer cooking. There are also good premade polentas available in the refrigerator section of most grocery stores that you can just slice, heat, and serve.

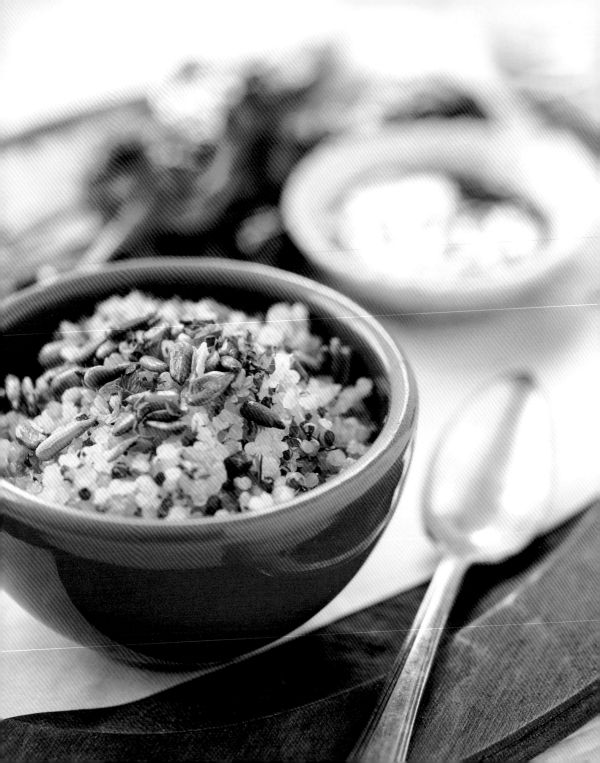

Quinoa Pilaf with Toasted Sunflower Seeds

Quinoa is a nutty, sweet, quick-cooking grain that is high in protein. It comes from the Andes Mountains of South America and was one of the three staple foods, along with corn and potatoes, of the Inca civilization. Quinoa was known then, and still is known in that area, as the mother grain.

MAKES 8 SERVINGS

1 cup quinoa
2¼ cups water
Pinch of sea salt

1 tablespoon sautéed onion (optional)
1 tablespoon toasted sunflower or
    sesame seeds (optional)

- Dry-roast the quinoa in a medium skillet over medium heat, stirring until golden.

- Bring the water and salt to a boil in a medium saucepan over medium heat. Add the quinoa and cover. Reduce the heat to medium-low and simmer for 20 minutes.

- Stir in the onion and sunflower seeds.

PER SERVING (½ cup): 169 calories, 4 g fat, 6 g protein, 27 g carbohydrates, 3 g fiber, 2 mg sodium

Spelt Pilaf with Baby Arugula

From Western Regional Executive Chef Charles Ramseyer,
China Grill Management

Spelt is an ancient European grain that is a distant cousin to modern wheat. It has a hearty, nutty flavor that has been popular in Italy for centuries.

MAKES 4 SERVINGS

1 cup spelt (or substitute kamut
    or farro)
2 tablespoons extra-virgin olive oil
2 cloves garlic, minced
2 shallots, finely chopped
1 small carrot, peeled and finely
    chopped
1 stalk celery, finely chopped

1 small bulb fennel, finely chopped
½ cup sauvignon blanc
1 to 2 cups chicken or vegetable stock
2 cups packed baby arugula,
    chopped
Kosher salt and freshly ground black
    pepper

> **♦ Nutrition Tip ♦**
>
> Spelt, kamut, and farro are forms of wheat. Kamut is an ancient Egyptian wheat, spelt is known as European wheat, while farro is Italian wheat. The three grains can be used interchangeably in recipes.

- Fill a 3-quart stockpot halfway with water (about 6 cups) and bring to a boil. Add the spelt and cook until al dente, about 20 minutes. Drain and set aside.

- Heat the oil in a medium saucepan over medium heat. Add the garlic, shallots, carrot, celery, and fennel. Sauté until the vegetables begin to soften.

- Add the wine and simmer until most of the liquid has evaporated. Add 1 cup of the stock and the cooked spelt. Simmer, adding more stock as needed, until the spelt is slightly chewy and has the consistency of risotto, about 20 minutes.

- Remove from the heat and stir in the arugula. Season to taste with salt and pepper and serve.

PER SERVING: 310 calories, 9 g fat, 8 g protein, 51 g carbohydrates, 3 g fiber, 922 mg sodium

Spanish Rice

From Jackie Patterson, cancer survivor

Color up your meal with this easy-to-prepare recipe that has excellent flavor.

MAKES 4 SERVINGS

2 cups water, or 1 cup low-sodium, nonfat chicken stock and 1 cup water
Kosher or sea salt
1 cup long-grain brown rice
One 15-ounce can stewed tomatoes

4 ounces turkey bacon, chopped
1 medium onion, chopped
1 small green bell pepper, chopped
2 tablespoons butter or no-trans-fat margarine

- Preheat the oven to 350 degrees F.

- Bring the water and a pinch of sea salt to a boil in a medium saucepan over medium heat. Add the rice and cover. Reduce the heat to medium-low and simmer undisturbed for 50 to 60 minutes.

> **♦ Contributor Tip ♦**
>
> You can cook once and eat four times by freezing single portions of this rice. Plus add steamed broccoli for your quota of greens.

- Drain the tomatoes, reserving the liquid, and chop them. Set aside.

- Fry the turkey bacon in a small skillet over medium heat. Transfer the bacon to a plate lined with paper towels to drain.

- Add the onion and pepper to the same pan, and sauté until the onion is transparent.

- Combine the rice, tomatoes with reserved liquid, bacon, sautéed onion mixture, and butter in a 2-quart casserole dish and stir well.

- Bake for 25 to 30 minutes and serve.

PER SERVING: 343 calories, 13 g fat, 10 g protein, 49 g carbohydrates, 5 g fiber, 773 mg sodium

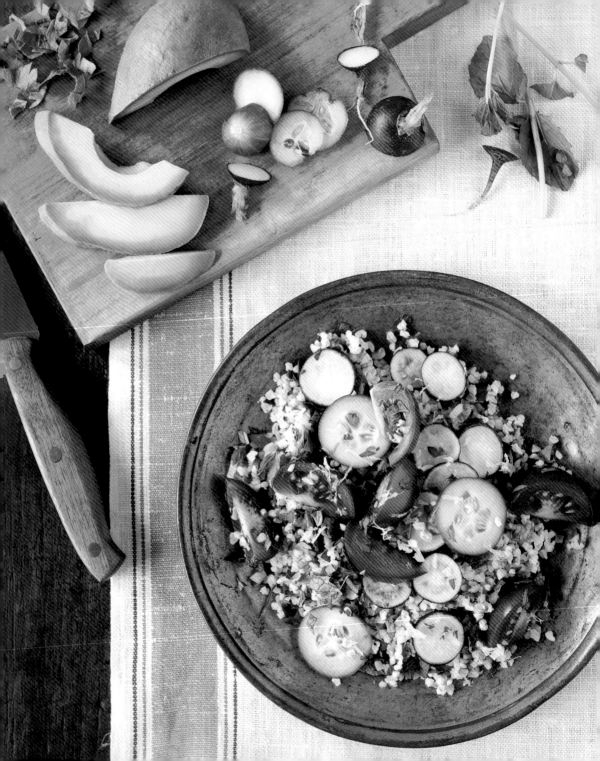

Tabouli

Tabouli is a traditional Middle Eastern salad made from bulgur wheat—wheat that has been precooked, cracked, and dried. Since it needs no further cooking, it's quick to whip up and ideal for summer days.

MAKES 3 SERVINGS

1 cup reduced-fat chicken or vegetable stock
1 cup bulgur wheat (tabouli)
1 tablespoon extra-virgin olive oil
½ cup chopped fresh parsley
2 tablespoons chopped fresh mint, basil, or cilantro
Juice from 1 medium lemon (about 3 tablespoons)

2 cloves garlic, minced
1 large tomato, chopped
½ avocado, cut into ½-inch-thick slices
½ cucumber, diced (optional)
6 radishes, diced (optional)
Grated zest of 1 lemon (optional)

• Bring the stock to a boil in a medium saucepan over medium heat. Add the bulgur. Return to a boil, then cover and remove from the heat.

• When the liquid has been absorbed, about 15 minutes, fluff the bulgur with a fork. Add the oil, parsley, mint, lemon juice, garlic, and tomato.

• Refrigerate until cool.

• Garnish with sliced avocado, cucumber, radishes, and lemon zest.

PER SERVING: 281 calories, 10 g fat, 8 g protein, 44 g carbohydrates, 11 g fiber, 28 mg sodium

♦ Cooking Tip ♦

Use more garlic and fresh mint in the recipe to add more bite and a breezy taste.

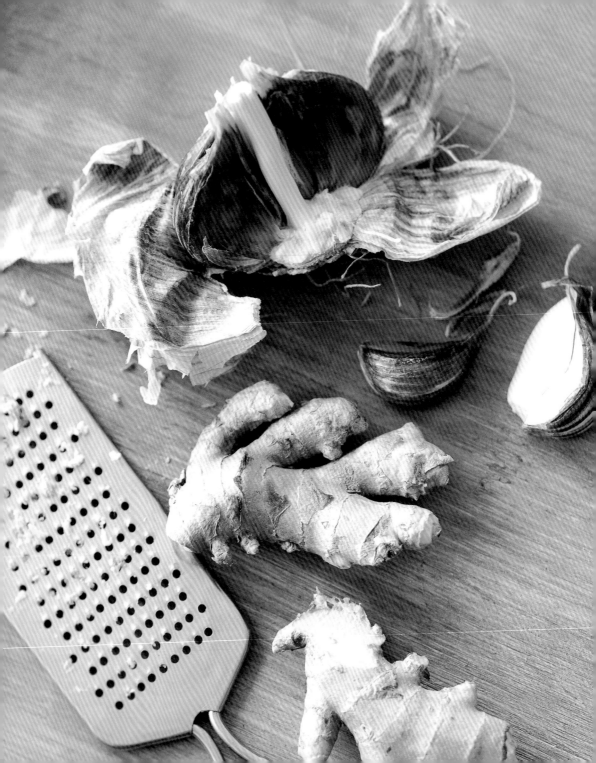

Entrées

Herb-Roasted Chicken 170

Pan-Seared Petrale Sole with
Lemon-Caper-Butter Sauce 171

Seattle Bouillabaisse 172

Stovetop Fish Stew with Gingered
Black Beans 174

Salmon with Sun-Dried
Tomato Sauce 175

Pizza with Sun-Dried
Tomato Sauce 178

Polenta Pizza 180

Potato Pancakes 181

Skillet Fajitas 183

Grilled Chicken Skewers with
Tangerine-Ginger Glaze 185

Easy Vegetable Stir-Fry with
Black Bean Sauce 188

Mushroom-Asparagus Stir-Fry
with Bay Scallops 189

Pork Yakisoba 190

Szechuan Stir-Fry 192

Broccoli and Lamb Stir-Fry with
Soy-Sherry Sauce 193

Spicy Miso Peanut Noodles 195

Basmati Rice with Lentils 196

Creamy Polenta and
Bean Casserole 197

Zucchini and Tomato Gratin 199

Spicy Chickpea, Kale, and
Tomato Stew 200

Hearty Greens and Grains with
Sesame Tofu Squares 202

Three-Bean Vegetarian Chili 205

Turkey Meat Loaf 206

Chicken Biscuit Pie 207

Cottage-Style Macaroni
and Cheese 209

Herb-Roasted Chicken

This full-flavored chicken is easy to prepare and makes a wonderful meal paired with Quinoa Pilaf with Toasted Sunflower Seeds, page 163, and a flavorful vegetable, like Honey-Glazed Green Beans with Almonds, page 147.

MAKES 4 TO 6 SERVINGS

One 3- to 4-pound whole frying or roasting chicken
1 small onion, peeled and halved
2 cloves garlic, smashed

1 teaspoon poultry seasoning
1 teaspoon curry powder (optional)
½ cup water or chicken stock, plus more for basting

- Preheat the oven to 400 degrees F.

- Remove the giblets and neck from the body cavity of the chicken. Rinse the chicken well and pat dry with paper towels. Stuff the cavity with the onion and garlic. Place the chicken, breast side up, in a roasting pan.

- Sprinkle the poultry seasoning and curry powder over the chicken and rub them in well. Add the water to the roasting pan.

- Cover the roasting pan with aluminum foil and cook for 30 minutes. Baste with the pan drippings, adding more water or stock as needed to keep the bird moist. Cook for another hour, basting as needed. Uncover the chicken for the last 15 minutes of cooking to brown the skin.

- Remove the skin before serving.

PER SERVING: 387 calories, 10 g fat, 68 g protein, 2 g carbohydrates, 0 g fiber, 246 mg sodium

> **• Nutrition Tip •**
>
> The skin of a chicken contains a large amount of fat. By removing the skin, the total fat intake is reduced from 47 grams to 10 grams of fat per serving.

Pan-Seared Petrale Sole with Lemon-Caper-Butter Sauce

From Chef Kaspar Donier, Kaspar's Special Events and Catering

MAKES 4 SERVINGS

3 tablespoons extra-virgin olive oil

Four 7-ounce petrale sole fillets

Kosher salt and freshly ground black pepper

Juice from 2 small lemons (about ¼ cup)

¼ cup sauvignon blanc

1½ teaspoons capers

3 tablespoons cold unsalted butter, cut into thin slices

1 tablespoon chopped fresh parsley

- Heat the oil in a 12-inch nonstick sauté pan over medium-high heat.

- Season the sole fillets to taste with salt and pepper.

- Place the fillets in the pan and sear until they begin to brown around the edges, 3 to 4 minutes. Turn and sear the other side for 1 minute. Carefully transfer the fillets to serving plates and keep warm.

- Add the lemon juice, wine, and capers to the same pan. Increase the heat to high and cook until the sauce boils vigorously. Reduce the heat to medium-high and add the butter, stirring or shaking the pan continuously until all the butter has melted and it has emulsified into a smooth sauce. Stir in the parsley and season to taste with salt and pepper.

- Top the fillets with the sauce and serve immediately.

PER SERVING: 366 calories, 21 g fat, 38 g protein, 2 g carbohydrates, 0 g fiber, 440 mg sodium

Seattle Bouillabaisse

Adapted from a recipe from Chef Greg Atkinson, Restaurant Marché, and author of At the Kitchen Table

Featuring a rich sauce of tomatoes, garlic, and kale, this hearty stew provides nutrition with flavor. Salmon fillets can be used in this recipe, but a white fish like halibut or snapper is more conventional. Add variety with shrimp, scallops, crab, or mussels. Or mix and match kale with mustard or collard greens.

MAKES 6 SERVINGS

¼ cup extra-virgin olive oil
2 medium onions, thinly sliced
2 tablespoons dried oregano
1 tablespoon dried basil
½ teaspoon dried thyme
½ teaspoon freshly ground
   black pepper
⅛ teaspoon cayenne pepper
   (optional)
¼ cup mild red wine vinegar

3 cups low-sodium vegetable broth
Generous pinch of saffron threads
2 tablespoons crushed garlic
One 22-ounce can low-sodium
   crushed Italian-style tomatoes
2 pounds fish fillets, or a combination
   of fish, shrimp, and scallops
1 large bunch kale, cut crosswise into
   fine ribbons (about 4 cups packed)

- Heat the oil in a large, heavy saucepan over medium-high heat. Sauté the onions until they just begin to brown. Stir in the oregano, basil, thyme, pepper, and cayenne.

- Add the vinegar and let the mixture boil until the vinegar has evaporated somewhat and the onions are frying again.

- Stir in the broth, saffron, and garlic and bring the mixture to a boil. Add the tomatoes. (The stew can be made ahead to this point and kept refrigerated until 20 minutes before serving time.)

- Bring the stew to a boil. Add the fish fillets and kale.

- Reduce the heat to low and simmer for 15 minutes. Serve immediately.

PER SERVING (1 cup): 370 calories, 16 g fat, 35 g protein,
19 g carbohydrates, 5 g fiber, 220 mg sodium

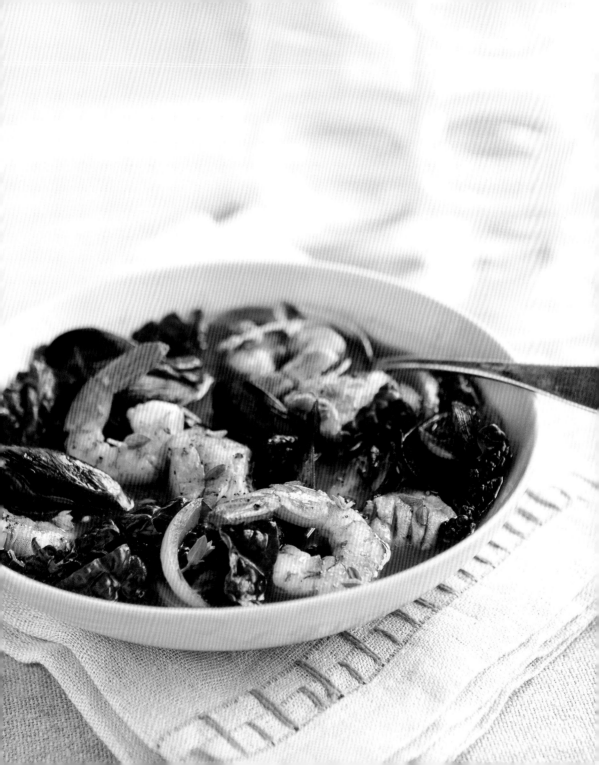

Stovetop Fish Stew with Gingered Black Beans

From Jeanne Ward, cancer survivor

This one-pot meal cooks in less than fifteen minutes.

MAKES 2 SERVINGS

2 tablespoons extra-virgin olive oil
1 medium onion, sliced
1 clove garlic, minced
1-inch piece fresh ginger, peeled and grated
One 8-ounce can low-sodium stewed tomatoes

One 16-ounce can low-sodium black beans, rinsed and drained
One 14-ounce halibut or other white fish fillet
Kosher or sea salt and freshly ground black pepper

- Heat the oil in a medium skillet over medium heat. Add the onion, garlic, and ginger and sauté until the onion is tender.

- Add the tomatoes and simmer for about 5 minutes. Add the black beans and stir well.

- Place the halibut on top of the bean mixture, and simmer until it flakes easily. Season to taste with salt and pepper.

- Serve the stew in bowls.

PER SERVING: 499 calories, 18 g fat, 34 g protein, 48 g carbohydrates, 16 g fiber, 1,130 mg sodium

Salmon with Sun-Dried Tomato Sauce

A variation on a Pacific Northwest favorite, inspired by the Greeks. This full-bodied, richly flavored tomato sauce complements a wide variety of dishes. Make the Pizza with Sun-Dried Tomato Sauce, page 178, for another way to use this sauce, or spoon it over tofu or vegetables.

MAKES 4 SERVINGS

¼ cup Sun-Dried Tomato Sauce (page 176)

Four 5-ounce salmon fillets

- Heat a large nonstick frying pan over medium-high heat. Put the tomato sauce in the pan.

- Place the salmon on top of the sauce, skin side down.

- Cook for 5 to 7 minutes. Turn the salmon over and continue cooking for another 5 minutes, or until it flakes easily.

PER SERVING (1 fillet): 269 calories, 16 g fat, 29 g protein, 1 g carbohydrates, 0 g fiber, 129 mg sodium

Sun-Dried Tomato Sauce

MAKES 2 CUPS

1 cup sun-dried tomatoes
3 large cloves garlic
1 cup boiling water
¼ cup fresh basil leaves
4 teaspoons fresh parsley leaves
1 tablespoon chopped shallot
Juice from ½ lemon (about
    1 tablespoon)

1 tablespoon red wine vinegar
1 teaspoon Dijon mustard
1 teaspoon low-sodium soy sauce
2 tablespoons extra-light olive oil
¼ teaspoon salt
¼ teaspoon crushed red pepper
    flakes

- Put the sun-dried tomatoes and garlic in a medium bowl and pour the boiling water over the top. Soak for 20 minutes.

- Place the basil, parsley, and shallot in a food processor and blend until very finely minced. Add the softened tomatoes and garlic and ½ cup of the soaking liquid. Blend thoroughly.

- Add the lemon juice, vinegar, mustard, soy sauce, oil, salt, and red pepper flakes. Blend until the sauce is a spreadable consistency, adding extra soaking liquid as needed.

PER SERVING (1 tablespoon): 27 calories, 2 g fat, 1 g protein, 2 g carbohydrates, 0 g fiber, 126 mg sodium

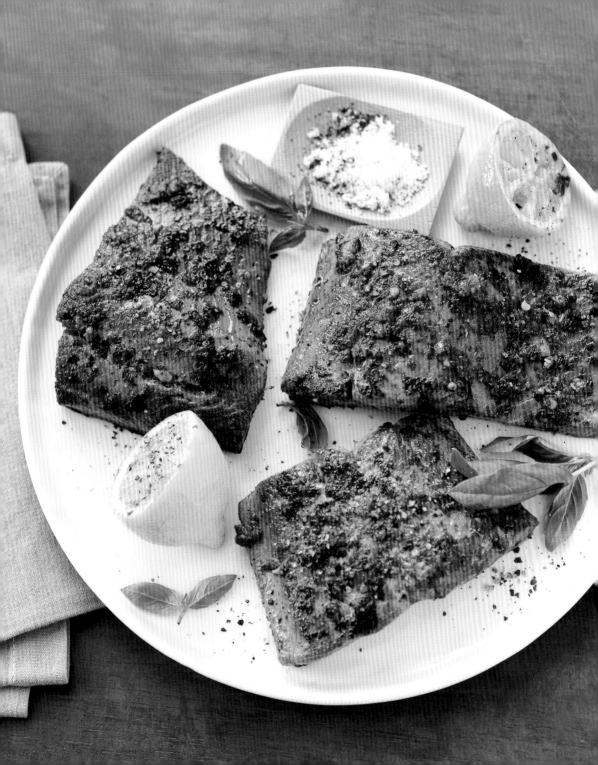

Pizza with Sun-Dried Tomato Sauce

This pizza is a delightful Sunday night treat that's bursting with flavor. Olives, zucchini, onions, tomatoes, anchovies, capers, or hot peppers may be added to suit individual tastes. The crust recipe makes enough for two 12-inch pizzas but it can easily be doubled and extra portions frozen for later use.

MAKES TWO 12-INCH PIZZAS

Crust
1 cup lukewarm water or milk
1 package active dry yeast
2 cups unbleached all-purpose flour
½ cup whole wheat pastry flour
½ teaspoon salt
1 tablespoon extra-virgin olive oil
Cornmeal

Sauce
Extra-virgin olive oil
2 cups tomato puree

¼ cup Sun-Dried Tomato Sauce
 (page 176)

Toppings
4 ounces part-skim mozzarella, grated
4 ounces part-skim ricotta cheese
8 cloves garlic, thinly sliced
Crushed dried red pepper
¼ teaspoon dried oregano
1 green bell pepper, sliced into
 thin rings
¼ pound mushrooms, thinly sliced

- To make the crust, pour the lukewarm water into a medium mixing bowl and sprinkle in the yeast. Let stand for 5 minutes, or until foamy.

- In a small bowl, combine the all-purpose and whole wheat flours.

- Add the salt, oil, and ½ cup of the combined flours to the mixing bowl. Stir briskly for several minutes with a wooden spoon.

- Add the remaining 2 cups combined flour, ½ cup at a time, mixing by hand after each addition. The dough should be a bit softer than bread dough but not as sticky.

- Turn the dough out onto a surface lightly dusted with cornmeal and knead for 5 minutes. Clean and oil the mixing bowl, and return the dough to the bowl. Set in a warm place (an unheated oven works well) for 30 to 45 minutes, or until the dough has risen and doubled in size. Note: If you're not proceeding with this recipe immediately, divide the dough in half and freeze it for later use (allowing 3 hours to thaw at room temperature).

- Preheat the oven to 500 degrees F and position a rack in the top third of the oven. Oil two 12-inch pizza pans.

- Punch the dough down, return it to a cornmeal-dusted surface, and knead for several minutes.

- Divide the dough in half and roll it out to fit the pans. Press the dough into place. Brush lightly with the oil. Spread the tomato puree and sun-dried tomato sauce over the pizzas.

- Cover with the cheeses and your choice of extra toppings.

- Bake each pizza on the top oven rack for 10 to 12 minutes, or until the crust is golden and the toppings are bubbling. Slice into 8 wedges and serve immediately.

PER SERVING (crust only; 1 slice): 257 calories, 7 g fat, 12 g protein, 40 g carbohydrates, 4 g fiber, 511 mg sodium

"Share your concerns, hopes, and joys with good friends who are fellow cancer patients or who have been touched by cancer."

—CLODAGH ASH, CANCER SURVIVOR

Polenta Pizza

An Italian dish that is simple to prepare yet achieves a sensational pizza-like result.

MAKES 8 SERVINGS

Crust
1 cup polenta
1½ cups low-sodium, low-fat
   chicken stock
1½ cups water
½ teaspoon salt
2 large eggs, beaten, at room
   temperature

Topping
1 tablespoon extra-virgin olive oil
½ cup diced onion
½ cup diced green bell pepper
½ cup diced red bell pepper
1 clove garlic, crushed
½ cup diced tomatoes
1 teaspoon dried oregano
1 cup grated part-skim mozzarella

♦ Cooking Tip ♦

This polenta pizza makes great leftovers for sack lunches.

- Preheat the oven to 350 degrees F. Spray a 9-inch pie pan with nonstick cooking spray.

- To make the crust, combine the polenta, stock, water, and salt in a medium saucepan over medium heat. Bring to a boil and simmer, stirring frequently, for about 10 minutes, or until thick. Remove from the heat and blend in the eggs, whisking constantly.

- Form the polenta into a thick crust in the pie pan. Let stand.

- To prepare the topping, heat the oil in a large skillet over medium heat. Sauté the onion, bell peppers, and garlic until tender. Remove from the heat and stir in the tomatoes and oregano.

- Spread the vegetable mixture over the polenta crust. Cover with the grated cheese. Bake for 45 minutes. Cut into 8 wedges and serve.

PER SERVING: 170 calories, 6 g fat, 8 g protein, 22 g carbohydrates, 3 g fiber, 310 mg sodium

Potato Pancakes

Recipes for potato pancakes vary only slightly, reflecting regional tastes. This version includes leeks and garlic and are baked, not fried. Serve with applesauce or low-fat sour cream. Potato pancakes make a fine accompaniment for meat, poultry, or fish.

MAKES 3 SERVINGS

1 large russet potato, peeled
   and grated
½ cup chopped leek or onion
2 tablespoons unbleached
   all-purpose flour

¼ teaspoon salt
½ clove garlic, chopped
2 egg whites, beaten
Extra-virgin olive oil

- Preheat the oven to 450 degrees F.

- In a mixing bowl, gently stir together the grated potato, leek, flour, salt, and garlic. Fold in the egg whites.

- Dot a baking sheet with ½ teaspoon oil and drop 1 tablespoon batter onto the oil. Repeat, spacing the pancakes 1 inch apart, until all the batter has been used.

- Bake for 15 minutes, or until golden brown. Turn the pancakes over and bake for another 10 minutes. Serve immediately.

PER SERVING: 84 calories, 1 g fat, 4 g protein, 15 g carbohydrates, 1 g fiber, 220 mg sodium

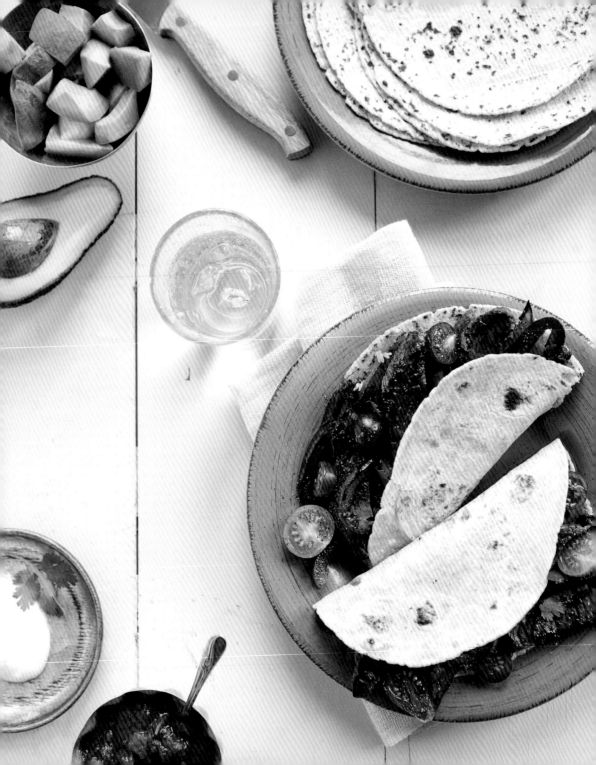

Skillet Fajitas

These tasty fajitas call for marinated flank steak, but you can substitute boneless, skinless chicken breasts; fish fillets; or a 10-ounce package of firm, silken-style light or reduced-fat tofu. As another alternative, try half tofu and half beef, chicken, or fish. Serve fajitas with nonfat refried beans, rice, or Texas Black Bean Salad, page 108.

MAKES 6 SERVINGS

¾ pound flank steak, cut into 1-inch strips
Citrus Marinade (page 184)
1 medium onion, sliced
1 green bell pepper, seeded and sliced into long, narrow strips
1 red bell pepper, seeded and sliced into long, narrow strips

3 cloves garlic, diced
6 whole wheat tortillas
2 tomatoes, chopped (optional)
Salsa (optional)
Minced cilantro (optional)
Chopped avocado (optional)
Plain nonfat yogurt or low-fat sour cream (optional)

- Preheat the oven to 350 degrees F.

- Put the steak strips in a medium bowl and cover with the citrus marinade. Let sit for at least 30 minutes, or longer for deeper flavor and more tender meat.

- Heat a nonstick skillet or wok over medium-high heat. Remove the steak from the marinade, add to the skillet, and stir-fry for 5 to 8 minutes. Add the onion, bell peppers, and garlic and stir-fry until just tender.

- Wrap the tortillas in aluminum foil and warm them in the oven for about 10 minutes.

- Fill each tortilla with an equal amount of meat and vegetables. Garnish with your choice of tomatoes, salsa, cilantro, avocado, and yogurt. Roll or fold the tortilla over the filling and serve.

PER SERVING: 308 calories, 9 g fat, 18 g protein, 39 g carbohydrates, 3 g fiber, 428 mg sodium

CITRUS MARINADE

This sensational, semisweet marinade enhances the flavor of chicken, fish, lean meat, tofu, or vegetables.

MAKES 2½ CUPS

Juice from 3 medium limes
(about ⅓ cup)
Juice from ½ lemon (about
1 tablespoon)
⅓ cup low-sodium soy sauce
2 tablespoons Worcestershire sauce
1 tablespoon Grand Marnier, plum
wine, sugar, or sherry

Juice from 3 medium oranges
(about 1 cup)
4 to 5 cloves garlic, pressed or
minced
½ cup chopped fresh cilantro
1-inch piece fresh ginger, peeled and
grated (optional)

• Combine all the ingredients in a medium bowl and stir well.

PER RECIPE: 266 calories, 1 g fat, 9 g protein, 55 g carbohydrates, 1 g fiber, 3,446 mg sodium

Grilled Chicken Skewers with Tangerine-Ginger Glaze

From Chef Tom Douglas, James Beard award winner and owner of ten Seattle restaurants

These flavorful skewers can be enjoyed as an appetizer or as a main course served with Brown Rice, page 158, and Garlic-Sautéed Greens, page 146.

MAKES 4 SERVINGS

1 cup freshly squeezed tangerine juice
½ cup mirin
¼ cup soy sauce
2 tablespoons firmly packed
   brown sugar
1 tablespoon granulated sugar
2 teaspoons grated fresh ginger
½ teaspoon chopped garlic
½ teaspoon grated tangerine zest

1 teaspoon cornstarch
1 teaspoon water
4 boneless, skinless chicken
   breast halves
16 bamboo skewers, soaked in
   water for 30 minutes
Peanut or vegetable oil
Kosher salt and freshly ground
   black pepper

- To make the tangerine-ginger glaze, combine the tangerine juice, mirin, soy sauce, brown and granulated sugars, ginger, garlic, and zest in a small saucepan over medium heat. Simmer until reduced by half, about 10 minutes.

- Make a slurry by mixing the cornstarch with the water in a small bowl. Add the slurry to the glaze and simmer for another minute. The glaze should be as thick as maple syrup. Reserve one-fourth of the glaze in a separate small bowl.

- Preheat a charcoal grill to medium heat or preheat the broiler.

- To prepare the chicken skewers, cut each chicken breast into 4 pieces about 2 inches long by 1 inch wide. Thread 1 piece of chicken onto each skewer, brush with the oil, and season to taste with salt and pepper.

continued

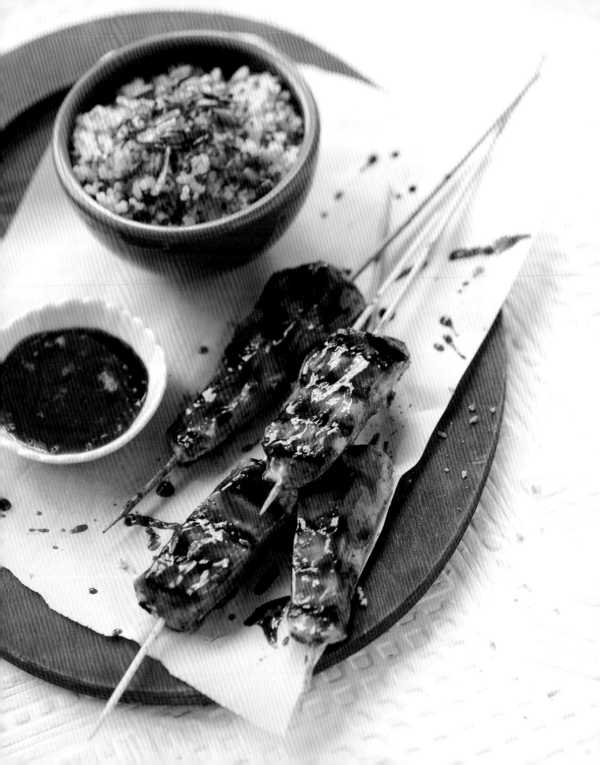

- Grill or broil the chicken skewers, turning them often and brushing 2 or 3 times with the glaze, until the chicken is cooked through, about 7 minutes. Watch carefully, since the sugars in the glaze can burn; adjust the distance from the heat as needed.

- Spoon the reserved glaze over the chicken just before serving.

PER SERVING (4 skewers): 306 calories, 5 g fat, 30 g protein, 27 g carbohydrates, 0 g fiber, 1,086 mg sodium

◆ Chef's Tip ◆

The tangerine glaze can be made a few days ahead and stored in an airtight container in the refrigerator. When chilled, the glaze will firm up. To smooth it out before brushing on the skewers, warm it over low heat, whisking occasionally.

Easy Vegetable Stir-Fry with Black Bean Sauce

A stir-fry with interesting flavors that can be varied with your choice of vegetables. Add chunks of firm tofu for extra protein. Serve with jasmine rice or Asian noodles.

MAKES 2 SERVINGS

1 tablespoon peanut oil
1 teaspoon chopped fresh ginger
1 teaspoon chopped garlic
One 16-ounce package fresh or frozen stir-fry vegetables
4 ounces chopped mushrooms
1 tablespoon low-sodium soy sauce
1 tablespoon black bean sauce

1 teaspoon Asian chili sauce
¼ cup low-sodium vegetable stock or water
1 teaspoon cornstarch
2 tablespoons water
2 teaspoons toasted sesame oil
¼ cup chopped green onions (optional)

• Heat the peanut oil in a wok or large skillet over medium-high heat. Add the ginger and garlic and stir-fry for 30 seconds. Add the vegetables, mushrooms, soy sauce, black bean sauce, chili sauce, and stock. Stir-fry for 3 minutes.

• Whisk the cornstarch with the water in a small bowl. Add to the stir-fry, along with the sesame oil. Toss well. Serve and garnish with green onions.

PER SERVING: 190 calories, 12 g fat, 7 g protein, 20 g carbohydrates, 6 g fiber, 480 mg sodium

> **• Cooking Tip •**
>
> Keep a variety of packaged stir-fry vegetables in your freezer for easy, last-minute meal preparation.

Mushroom-Asparagus Stir-Fry with Bay Scallops

Mushrooms are one of our Top 10 "Super Foods." This recipe showcases this versatile ingredient alongside asparagus and bay scallops.

MAKES 4 TO 6 SERVINGS

3 tablespoons low-sodium soy sauce

1 teaspoon cornstarch

2 tablespoons sesame oil

6 asparagus spears, trimmed and cut into 1-inch pieces

6 shiitake or button mushrooms, sliced

3 green onions (green and white parts), sliced (or substitute 1 medium leek, white and light green parts only)

1 medium carrot, peeled and sliced

½ red bell pepper, cut into matchstick pieces

1 zucchini, sliced

3 large cloves garlic, finely chopped

2 teaspoons minced fresh ginger

½ pound fresh or thawed frozen bay scallops

• Combine the soy sauce and cornstarch in a small bowl.

• Lightly coat a nonstick skillet or wok with the oil. Place over high heat. Add the asparagus, mushrooms, onions, carrot, bell pepper, zucchini, garlic, and ginger. Stir-fry for about 8 minutes.

• Add the scallops and cook for 6 minutes, or until the vegetables are tender and the scallops are white throughout.

• Stir in the soy sauce mixture and cook for 1 minute, or until thickened. Serve immediately.

PER SERVING: 128 calories, 6 g fat, 10 g protein, 9 g carbohydrates, 2 g fiber, 443 mg sodium

Pork Yakisoba

Adapted from a recipe by Mark Bittman, author and New York Times food journalist

This skillet meal combines just the right flavors, colors, and textures of vegetables with tender pork and noodles in a tangy sauce. Serve as a complete meal and enjoy leftovers for lunch or a snack the next day.

MAKES 8 SERVINGS

1 teaspoon salt
6 ounces soba noodles
1 tablespoon sesame oil
2 tablespoons organic canola oil or peanut oil
2 tablespoons minced ginger
2 pork chops, thinly sliced
2 carrots, shredded (about 2 cups)
½ medium cabbage, shredded (about 4 cups)
½ medium onion, thinly sliced (about 1 cup)
2 cups broccoli florets and stems
¼ cup low-sodium soy sauce
¼ cup Worcestershire sauce
2 teaspoons sugar
2 tablespoons rice vinegar
1 bunch scallions, chopped

- Bring a pot of water and the salt to a boil. Add the soba noodles and cook until al dente following the manufacturer's directions. Drain, transfer the noodles to a medium bowl, and stir in the sesame oil to prevent sticking.

- Heat the canola oil in a large skillet over medium-high heat. Add the ginger and cook for about 1 minute. Add pork and cook until evenly browned.

- Add the carrots, cabbage, onion, and broccoli to the skillet. Cook, stirring occasionally, until the vegetables are tender, adding water as needed.

- In a separate bowl, whisk together the soy sauce, Worcestershire, sugar, and rice vinegar.

- Add the noodles and sauce to the skillet and toss well to coat the vegetables and noodles. Garnish with the scallions.

PER SERVING (1 cup): 222 calories, 9 g fat, 21 g protein, 17 g carbohydrates, 3 g fiber, 451 mg sodium

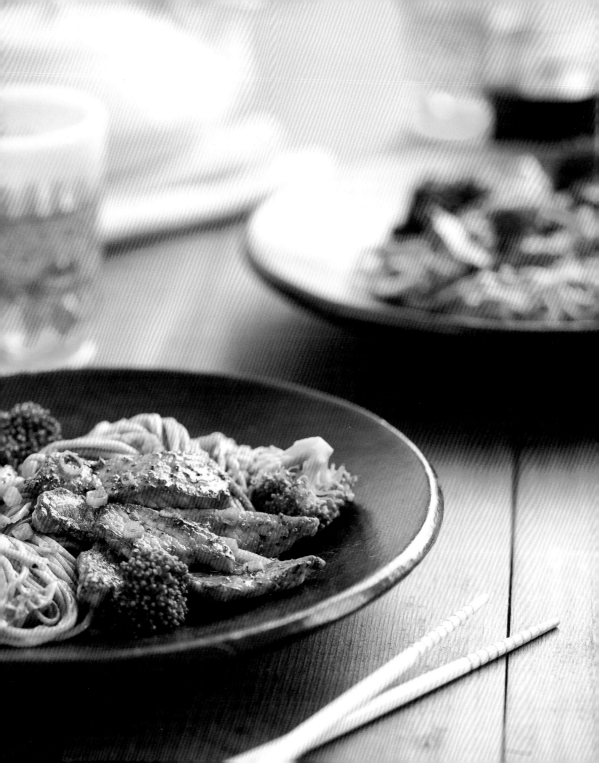

Szechuan Stir-Fry

Serve this tasty entrée with Brown Rice, page 158, or jasmine rice. It comes together very quickly.

MAKES 4 SERVINGS

One 16-ounce package extra-firm
    tofu, drained and patted dry
4 tablespoons peanut oil, divided
2 small zucchini, roughly chopped
    (about 1 cup)
½ yellow bell pepper, roughly
    chopped (about 1 cup)

3 small carrots, roughly chopped
    (about 1 cup)
½ small onion, roughly chopped
    (about 1 cup)
Szechuan Sauce (recipe follows)
⅓ cup roasted unsalted peanuts

♦ Chef's Note ♦

If you can't find roasted unsalted peanuts, you can rinse the salt off before adding them to the stir-fry.

- Preheat the oven to 450 degrees F.

- Chop the tofu into 1-inch cubes and put in a medium bowl. Add 2 tablespoons of the oil and toss well to coat. Spread the tofu on a baking sheet, and bake for 20 to 25 minutes, or until golden brown.

- Heat the remaining 2 tablespoons oil in a wok over medium-high heat. Add the tofu, zucchini, bell pepper, carrots, onion, and Szechuan sauce and stir-fry for 4 to 5 minutes, or until the vegetables are tender. Add the peanuts and stir for another minute to combine the flavors. Serve immediately.

PER SERVING: 419 calories, 29 g fat, 16 g protein, 29 g carbohydrates, 4 g fiber, 482 mg sodium

SZECHUAN SAUCE

¼ cup hoisin sauce
¼ cup dry sherry, white wine, or water
2 tablespoons minced garlic
2 tablespoons minced fresh ginger

1 tablespoon low-sodium soy sauce
½ to 1 teaspoon Asian chili sauce
½ teaspoon Szechuan peppercorns,
    crushed

- Whisk together all the ingredients in a medium bowl.

Broccoli and Lamb Stir-Fry with Soy-Sherry Sauce

Serve with jasmine rice or Asian noodles.

MAKES 4 SERVINGS

Garlic-Ginger Marinade (page 194)
1 pound leg of lamb or loin meat, cut
  into thin strips
2 cups broccoli florets
2 tablespoons peanut oil

2 cloves garlic, minced
Soy-Sherry Sauce (page 194)
1 tablespoon cornstarch (optional)
2 to 3 tablespoons water (optional)

• Put the marinade in a shallow dish and add the lamb. Refrigerate for
  20 minutes.

• Meanwhile, bring a medium pot of salted water to a boil, and blanch the broccoli for 2 minutes. Plunge into cold water. Drain and set aside.

• Heat 1 tablespoon of the oil in a wok over medium-high heat. Remove the
  lamb from the marinade, add to the wok, and stir-fry for 1 minute. Transfer
  the lamb to a bowl.

• Heat the remaining 1 tablespoon oil in the wok. Add the garlic and broccoli
  and stir-fry for 30 seconds. Return the lamb to the wok and pour in the soy-
  sherry sauce. Bring to a boil.

• In a small bowl, mix the cornstarch and water. Stir it into the sauce to thicken.
  Serve immediately.

PER SERVING: 352 calories, 24 g fat, 21 g protein, 12 g
carbohydrates, 1 g fiber, 1,067 mg sodium

Garlic-Ginger Marinade

2 tablespoons oyster sauce
2 tablespoons low-sodium soy sauce
2 tablespoons cornstarch

1 tablespoon dry sherry
1 tablespoon minced fresh ginger
2 cloves garlic, minced

• In a medium bowl, whisk together all the ingredients.

Soy-Sherry Sauce

¼ cup chicken stock
2 tablespoons low-sodium soy sauce
2 tablespoons sherry vinegar

1 teaspoon toasted sesame oil
1 teaspoon Asian chili sauce
1 tablespoon minced cilantro

• In a small bowl, whisk together all the ingredients.

Spicy Miso Peanut Noodles

From Chef Seppo Ed Farrey, author of 3 Bowls: Vegetarian Recipes from an
American Zen Buddhist Monastery

Serve this fun noodle dish with Garlic-Sautéed Greens, page 146, on the side.

MAKES 4 TO 6 SERVINGS

1 pound spaghetti, buckwheat, or
  other noodles
2 large carrots, peeled and coarsely
  grated
6 green onions (green and white
  parts), thinly sliced

2 medium red bell peppers, cut into
  1-inch slivers
Peanut Sauce (recipe follows)
3 tablespoons sesame seeds,
  toasted, for garnish (optional)

• In a large pot, cook the spaghetti according to package directions. Drain well.
  Rinse with cold water and drain again.

• Reserving a small amount of each vegetable for garnish, in a large bowl, toss
  the carrots, green onions, and bell peppers with the noodles and peanut sauce.
  Garnish with the reserved vegetables and sesame seeds.

PER SERVING: 593 calories, 20 g fat, 21 g protein, 86 g
carbohydrates, 6 g fiber, 788 mg sodium

PEANUT SAUCE

¾ cup smooth peanut butter
¾ cup hot water
½ cup white miso
¼ cup honey

2 tablespoons apple cider vinegar
1 tablespoon grated fresh ginger
½ teaspoon cayenne pepper
2 cloves garlic, minced

• In a medium bowl, whisk together all the ingredients until well combined. The
  sauce should take on a glossy sheen.

Basmati Rice with Lentils

This is a super simple one-pot meal that comes together in a flash. Serve with a salad of baby greens and crusty whole grain bread.

MAKES 2 SERVINGS

2 cups water
1½ cups low-sodium, nonfat
   chicken stock
1 small onion, diced
2 cloves garlic, diced
2 carrots, peeled and sliced

¼ teaspoon ground white pepper
½ teaspoon ground cumin
½ cup basmati rice
½ cup dried lentils, picked over
   and rinsed

- In a large pan, combine the water, stock, onion, garlic, carrots, white pepper, and cumin. Bring to a boil over medium-high heat. Slowly stir in the rice and lentils and return to a boil.

- Cover and reduce the heat to low. Simmer for 45 minutes, or until the lentils and rice are tender.

PER SERVING: 420 calories, 3 g fat, 23 g protein, 80 g carbohydrates, 18 g fiber, 160 mg sodium

◆ Cooking Tip ◆

Peel onions under cold water. The water rinses away the volatile sulfur that causes teary eyes. Or freeze the onion for 20 minutes before chopping.

Creamy Polenta and Bean Casserole

Here is a satisfying meal that features a winning combination of fiber-rich plant protein, whole grains, and chicken flavor. Serve with a vegetable dish such as Ruby Chard with Garlic, Chile, and Lemon, page 145, or a green salad such as Spinach Salad with Poppy Seed Balsamic Vinaigrette, page 106.

MAKES 4 SERVINGS

2 cups plus 2 tablespoons low-sodium chicken stock
1 cup polenta
⅓ cup grated part-skim mozzarella
1 skinless, boneless chicken breast, cut into 1-inch cubes
½ cup chopped onion

2 cloves garlic, minced or pressed
½ teaspoon ground cumin
½ cup salsa
One 15-ounce can low-sodium black, white, or kidney beans or black-eyed peas, rinsed and drained

- Preheat the oven to 350 degrees F.

- Combine 2 cups of the stock and the polenta in a medium saucepan over medium heat. Bring to a boil and cook, stirring constantly, until thick and smooth, about 5 minutes. Remove from the heat. Stir in the cheese and allow the polenta to cool.

- Meanwhile, in a medium skillet over medium heat, cook the chicken in the remaining 2 tablespoons stock for about 10 minutes, or until cooked through. Add the onion and garlic and cook until softened. Stir in the cumin, salsa, and beans.

- Spread the cooled polenta in the bottom of a nonstick 9-by-13-inch baking dish. Spoon the chicken and beans over the top.

- Bake for 20 minutes and serve.

PER SERVING: 356 calories, 5 g fat, 28 g protein, 49 g carbohydrates, 7 g fiber, 647 mg sodium

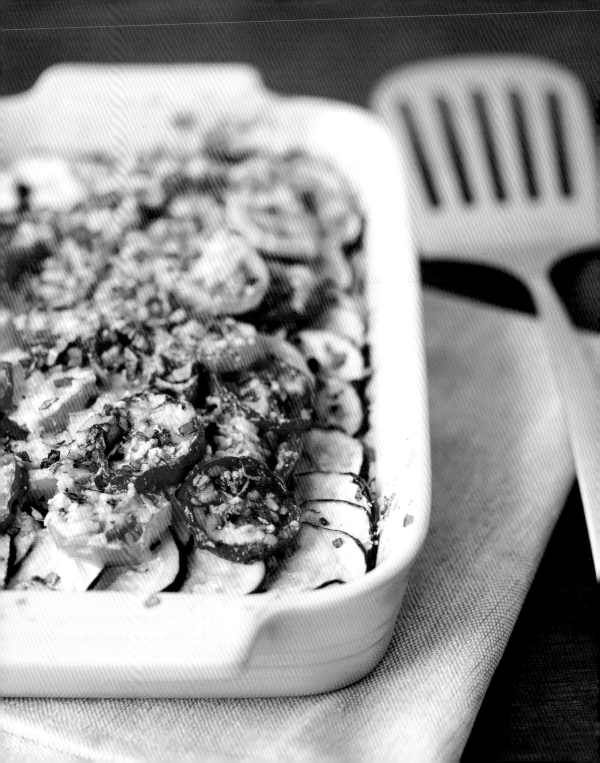

Zucchini and Tomato Gratin

This gratin is a delicious way to eat your vegetables.

MAKES 4 SERVINGS

1 tablespoon extra-virgin olive oil
2 cloves garlic, minced
2 tablespoons finely chopped onion
2 fresh basil leaves, chopped
½ cup white rice
2 small zucchini, sliced ¼ inch thick

4 medium tomatoes, sliced ½ inch thick
1 cup boiling water
Salt and freshly ground black pepper
½ cup grated Asiago cheese, or ¼ cup
　grated Parmesan or Romano (using
　less of these still gives ample flavor)

+ Preheat the oven to 375 degrees F.

+ Put the oil in an 8-inch square baking dish and spread to coat the bottom. Sprinkle the garlic, onion, and basil over the oil. Spread the rice over the top.

+ Layer the zucchini and tomato slices over the rice, and pour the boiling water over the top. Season with salt and pepper.

+ Bake for 20 minutes. Sprinkle the cheese over the top and bake for another 10 to 15 minutes, or until the cheese is golden brown and the vegetables and rice are cooked. Serve immediately.

PER SERVING: 198 calories, 8 g fat, 7 g protein, 26 g carbohydrates, 2 g fiber, 50 mg sodium

Spicy Chickpea, Kale, and Tomato Stew

From Julie Hillers, cancer survivor

Add spice to your life with this flavorful stew that combines the colors of golden curry with green kale, red tomatoes, and brown mushrooms. The bonus is that they are cancer-fighting "super foods" too. Serve with Quinoa Pilaf with Toasted Sunflower Seeds, page 163, for a nourishing meal.

MAKES 4 SERVINGS

2 tablespoons extra-virgin olive oil
½ onion, chopped
2 cloves garlic, minced
1 medium boneless, skinless chicken breast, chopped into 1-inch pieces (optional)
Spice mix of your choice, see box on page 201
One 15.5-ounce can low-sodium garbanzo beans, rinsed and drained

One 14.5-ounce can low-sodium chopped tomatoes with their juices
1 cup chicken broth, vegetable broth, or water
1 red bell pepper, chopped (about 1 cup)
8 white mushrooms, chopped into ½-inch pieces
1 bunch kale, stems removed and leaves chopped (about 4 cups), or 2 cups chopped spinach

• Heat the oil in a large saucepan over medium heat. Add the onion and cook, stirring occasionally, for 3 to 5 minutes, or until slightly browned. Add the garlic and chicken and cook for about 5 minutes, or until the chicken has turned white.

♦ Contributor's Note ♦

This recipe is very flexible and can easily adapt to what you like and what's in your pantry. For example, you can add potatoes or sweet potatoes. Chop them into ½-inch cubes and add with the bell pepper and mushrooms. Simmer the stew for a little longer, until the potatoes are fork-tender.

- Meanwhile, combine the spices of choice in a small bowl and stir well.

- Add the garbanzo beans, tomatoes with juices, broth, bell pepper, and mushrooms to the pan. Increase the heat to medium-high, stir in the spices, and stir occasionally until the mixture comes to a boil.

- Reduce the heat to medium-low, cover the pan, and let the stew simmer for 10 minutes. Add the kale, stirring to submerge it in the stew, cover, and simmer for 5 more minutes.

- Taste to adjust the seasonings; curry powders vary in their flavor and heat, so add more curry powder or red pepper flakes as desired. Serve hot.

PER SERVING: 321 calories, 9 g fat, 24 g protein, 37 g carbohydrates, 8 g fiber, 888 mg sodium

◆ Spice Mixes ◆

MILD: 2 teaspoons curry power, ½ teaspoon salt, ¼ teaspoon freshly ground black pepper

MEDIUM: 3 teaspoons curry powder, ¼ teaspoon crushed red pepper flakes, ½ teaspoon salt, ¼ teaspoon freshly ground black pepper

SPICY: 3 to 4 teaspoons curry powder, ½ teaspoon crushed red pepper flakes, ½ teaspoon salt, ¼ teaspoon freshly ground black pepper

Hearty Greens and Grains with Sesame Tofu Squares

Tofu, quinoa, amaranth, chard, spinach, and sesame seeds are all rich sources of calcium. The nutrients in this fun-to-assemble dish offer support and protection for the body during times of transition and stress.

MAKES 4 SERVINGS

One 16-ounce package firm tofu, or prebaked or seasoned tofu
2 cups plus 3 tablespoons water, divided
1 cup quinoa or amaranth, or a combination
1½ pounds chard, spinach, kale, or other greens, chopped

¼ cup sesame seeds, toasted
2 tablespoons low-sodium soy sauce, plus additional for serving
2 tablespoons minced fresh ginger
2 tablespoons minced garlic
Freshly squeezed lemon juice or rice vinegar, for serving (optional)

• Drain the tofu, slice into bars, and lay them over paper towels to drain off moisture. You may have to do this several times (removing soaked paper towels and laying down dry ones) so that the tofu will hold its texture and absorb flavors. Cut the bars into cubes.

• Bring 2 cups of the water to a boil in a medium saucepan over medium heat. Stir in the quinoa. Reduce the heat to low, cover, and cook until the liquid is absorbed and the quinoa is tender, about 20 minutes.

• Place chard in a steamer basket over boiling water. Steam the greens just until wilted. Set aside.

• Place the sesame seeds in a shallow bowl and gently roll the tofu cubes in them to coat on all sides.

continued

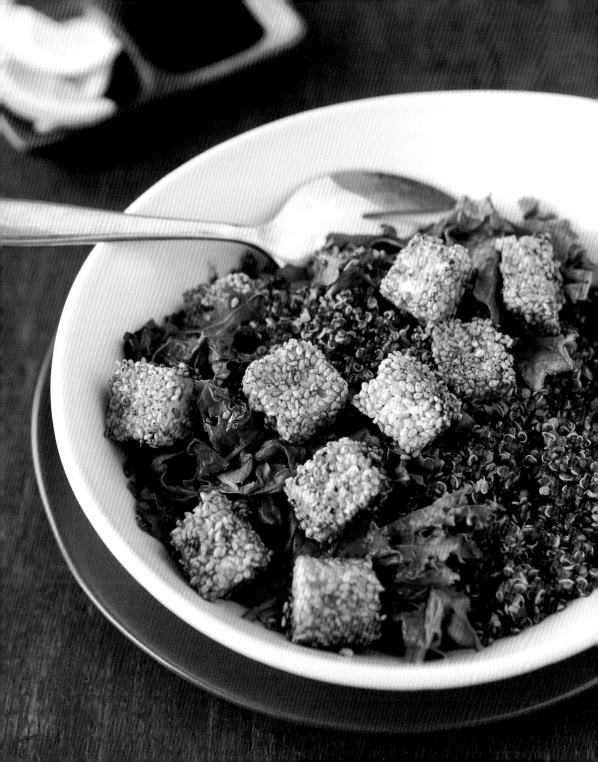

- In a large nonstick skillet, heat the soy sauce and remaining 3 tablespoons water. Add the ginger and garlic and sauté for 2 minutes. Add the sesame-coated tofu cubes. Cook, turning occasionally, for 5 to 7 minutes.

- Fluff the quinoa with a fork and divide among 4 serving bowls. Place the greens over the quinoa and top with the tofu. Serve with additional soy sauce and lemon juice or rice vinegar.

PER SERVING: 588 calories, 19 g fat, 36 g protein, 77 g carbohydrates, 13 g fiber, 696 mg sodium

> **Cooking tip from recipe tester Sara Snyder:**
> "I used amaranth and kale for this great recipe. I also deviated from it slightly by using some medium tofu, and I really liked how the softer texture sort of melted in your mouth. Also, I suggest adding a little fresh lemon juice."

Three-Bean Vegetarian Chili

This hearty chili can be served on a bed of rice, and Quick Corn Bread, page 155, makes a perfect accompaniment. For extra protein, cut firm tofu into ½-inch cubes and add just before the hot chiles.

MAKES 6 SERVINGS

2 tablespoons extra-virgin olive oil
½ cup chopped onion
4 cloves garlic, minced
1 green bell pepper, diced
1 zucchini, diced
2 tablespoons chili powder
1 teaspoon ground cumin
1 teaspoon dried oregano

One 15-ounce can low-sodium pinto beans
One 15-ounce can low-sodium black beans
Half 15-ounce can low-sodium garbanzo beans
One 15-ounce can tomato sauce
Hot chiles, chopped
Grated cheddar cheese

• Heat the oil in a Dutch oven or large saucepan over medium heat. Add the onion, garlic, bell pepper, and zucchini and sauté for 5 minutes.

• Add the chili powder, cumin, oregano, beans, and tomato sauce. Simmer for 30 minutes to combine the flavors. Season to taste with hot chiles.

• Serve in bowls with a sprinkling of cheese.

PER SERVING: 338 calories, 7 g fat, 17 g protein, 55 g carbohydrates, 17 g fiber, 500 mg sodium

Turkey Meat Loaf

A new twist on an all-American favorite. Substituting ground turkey for the traditional ground beef helps to significantly reduce the fat content. Steamed vegetables such as potatoes, carrots, turnips, or rutabagas make a fine accompaniment.

MAKES 6 SERVINGS

1 pound ground turkey breast, or ½ pound ground turkey and one 10-ounce package tofu, drained
1 medium onion, chopped
2 cloves garlic, diced
1 medium carrot, peeled and coarsely grated

½ cup rolled oats, quick-cooking or regular
2 large eggs
Half 14-ounce can low-sodium stewed tomatoes, chopped or coarsely pureed
⅛ teaspoon freshly ground black pepper (optional)

- Preheat the oven to 350 degrees F.

- Mix the turkey in a large bowl with the onion, garlic, carrot, oats, and eggs. Add the chopped tomatoes and pepper and stir well.

- Shape the mixture into a loaf and transfer to a 9-by-5-inch loaf pan.

- Cover the loaf with aluminum foil and bake for 60 minutes. Remove the foil and cook for about 15 minutes more, or until browned. Check that the internal temperature is 160 degrees F.

- Let stand 10 minutes before cutting into slices to serve.

PER SERVING (1 slice): 219 calories, 9 g fat, 19 g protein, 15 g carbohydrates, 3 g fiber, 125 mg sodium

Chicken Biscuit Pie

This is a "heritage" recipe: soul satisfying and hearty. Leftover cooked chicken or turkey may be substituted for the chicken breasts.

MAKES 8 SERVINGS

Two 15-ounce cans low-sodium chicken broth, divided
3 cups boneless, skinless chicken breast, sliced
1 medium red potato, diced
1 stalk celery, chopped
½ cup chopped red bell pepper
2 cloves garlic, minced
2 medium carrots, thinly sliced
1 small leek, chopped
1 cup sliced fresh mushrooms

One 15-ounce can no-sugar-added peas
¼ cup unbleached all-purpose flour
2 tablespoons whole wheat pastry flour
½ teaspoon poultry seasoning
¼ teaspoon freshly ground black pepper
1 cup low-fat milk
Biscuit Topping (recipe follows)

- Preheat the oven to 400 degrees F.

- Heat ¼ cup of the broth in a medium nonstick skillet over medium heat. Add the chicken and sauté for 10 minutes, or until cooked through. Transfer to a bowl and set side.

- Bring the remaining broth to a boil in a large saucepan over medium-high heat. Add the potato, celery, bell pepper, and garlic. Cover and cook for 5 minutes. Add the carrots and leek and simmer for 3 minutes. Add the mushrooms and peas and cook for 5 more minutes, or until all the vegetables are tender. Reduce the heat to medium.

- In a small bowl, combine the all-purpose and whole wheat flours, poultry seasoning, and pepper. Whisk in the milk. Pour into the saucepan with the

continued

vegetables and cook, stirring constantly, for 3 minutes, or until the gravy is thickened and bubbly. Remove from the heat and stir in the cooked chicken.

• Transfer the chicken and vegetables to a nonstick 9-by-13-inch baking dish. Using a large tablespoon, drop 16 spoonfuls of biscuit topping evenly over the top of the filling. Bake for about 28 minutes, or until the biscuit topping is golden brown.

PER SERVING: 304 calories, 7 g fat, 24 g protein, 35 g carbohydrates, 3 g fiber, 412 mg sodium

BISCUIT TOPPING

1 cup unbleached all-purpose flour
1 cup whole wheat pastry flour
2 teaspoons baking powder

½ teaspoon salt
1 cup nonfat milk or buttermilk
1 tablespoon butter, melted

• Combine the all-purpose and whole wheat flours, baking powder, and salt in a medium bowl and mix well. Stir in the milk and butter until the mixture forms a moist, loose dough.

• Set aside until ready to bake.

> **Cooking tip from recipe tester Justin:** "Although the recipe looked complicated, I ended up organizing my kitchen so that I chopped up certain items that would be added together and put them into individual bowls together so I could easily do a step-by-step following of the recipe."

Cottage-Style Macaroni and Cheese

From Merrilee Buckley, former Cancer Lifeline intern

Comfort food with a twist, this mac and cheese really delivers in the flavor department. For a smoother texture, puree the cottage cheese and milk in a blender before adding to the sauce.

MAKES 4 SERVINGS

2 cups whole wheat elbow macaroni
1 cup low-fat cottage cheese
1½ cups grated reduced-fat sharp or
   extra-sharp cheddar cheese
½ cup reduced-fat milk
½ onion, minced or pulsed in a food
   processor
Salt and freshly ground black pepper

- Preheat the oven to 350 degrees F.

- In a large pot, cook the macaroni according to package directions. Drain.

- Put the macaroni in a mixing bowl. Add the cottage cheese, cheddar, milk, onion, and salt and pepper to taste. Mix well.

- Transfer the macaroni to a baking dish and bake for about 30 minutes, or until the cheese is completely melted.

PER SERVING: 374 calories, 11 g fat, 27 g protein, 48 g carbohydrates, 5 g fiber, 251 mg sodium

◆ Cooking Tip ◆

You can add ¼ cup grated Parmesan cheese to this recipe for extra flavor.

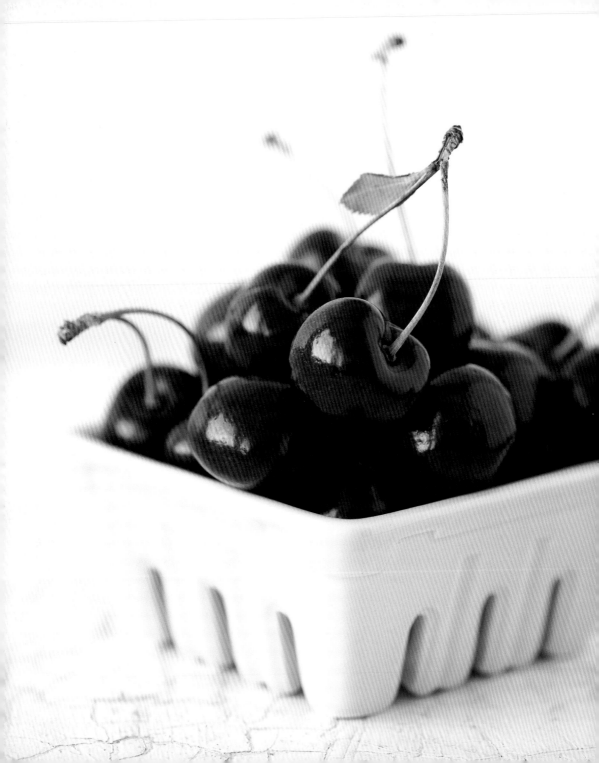

Desserts

Almond-Crusted Pears in Orange Sauce

A refreshing dessert that is easy to prepare, yet special enough for company.

MAKES 2 SERVINGS

Juice from ½ lemon (about
  2 teaspoons)
Juice from 1 small orange (about
  ¼ cup)
1 tablespoon sugar

1½ teaspoons cornstarch
Zest from ½ small orange (about
  1 teaspoon)
1 pear, cored and sliced into 6 wedges
2 tablespoons chopped almonds

- In a small saucepan, combine the lemon and orange juices, sugar, cornstarch, and orange zest and cook over medium heat until thick, stirring constantly.

- Arrange the pear slices on 2 serving plates. Pour the sauce evenly over the pear slices. Sprinkle with the chopped almonds and chill until ready to serve.

PER SERVING: 97 calories, 0 g fat, 1 g protein, 25 g carbohydrates, 2 g fiber, 1 mg sodium

◆ Cooking Tip ◆

To save your energy, buy nuts already chopped.
Extra nuts can be stored in airtight containers
in the refrigerator for 2 to 3 weeks and will keep
almost indefinitely in the freezer.

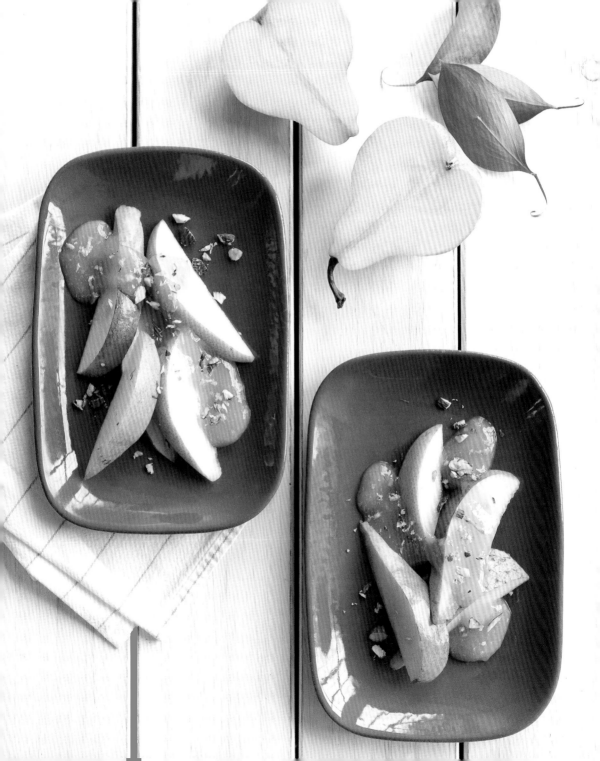

Pecan Honey-Baked Apples

This dessert is a delicious way to get a serving of fruit, with a satisfying, protein-rich addition of pecans.

MAKES 4 SERVINGS

4 large baking apples
¼ cup chopped pecans
¼ cup raisins
¼ to ½ cup honey

2 teaspoons butter or no-trans-fat
  margarine
¾ cup boiling water

- Preheat the oven to 375 degrees F.

- Wash the apples and remove the cores to within ½ inch of the bottoms. Cut a strip of peel from around the top of each apple.

- Fill each apple with 1 tablespoon each pecans and raisins. Drizzle 1 to 2 tablespoons of honey over the nuts and raisins in each apple and dab ½ teaspoon of butter on top.

- Place the apples in an 8-inch square baking dish and pour the boiling water into the dish. Bake for 40 to 60 minutes, or until the apples are tender. Baste with the pan juices and serve.

PER SERVING (1 apple): 257 calories, 7 g fat, 1 g protein, 53 g carbohydrates, 5 g fiber, 8 mg sodium

Raisin-Apple-Date Cookies

From Susan Hodges, author of Healthy Snacks

The sweetness of three rich fruits combines to make a cookie that tastes so good you won't miss the absence of added sugars.

MAKES 4 DOZEN COOKIES

1 cup raisins
½ cup chopped dates
1 cup peeled, sliced apple
1 cup apple juice concentrate
¼ cup (½ stick) butter or no-trans-fat
   margarine, at room temperature
2 egg whites

1 teaspoon vanilla extract
2 cups whole wheat flour
1 teaspoon baking soda
1 cup rolled oats (regular or
   quick-cooking)
½ cup chopped walnuts

• Preheat the oven to 350 degrees F. Line a baking sheet with parchment paper or spray with nonstick cooking spray.

• In a medium saucepan, combine the raisins, dates, apple slices, and apple juice concentrate. Bring to a boil and cook for 10 minutes.

• Stir the butter into the hot mixture. Allow to cool.

• Pour the mixture into a large mixing bowl. Add the egg whites and vanilla. Beat well. Stir in the flour, baking soda, and oats. Add the walnuts.

• Drop by teaspoonfuls onto the prepared baking sheet. Bake for 15 minutes, or until lightly browned.

PER SERVING (1 cookie): 74 calories, 2 g fat, 2 g protein, 13 g carbohydrates, 1 g fiber, 40 mg sodium

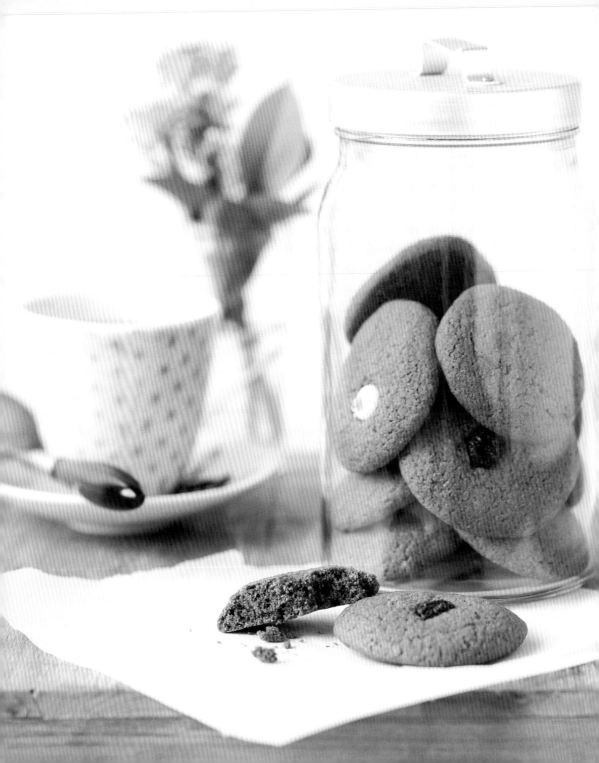

Gingerbread Molasses Cookies

From Chef Cynthia Lair, excerpted from her book Feeding the Young Athlete

Molasses gives these cookies an appealing sweetness with a touch of tangy ginger. If you can't find teff flour, just substitute an equal amount of additional whole wheat pastry flour.

MAKES 2 DOZEN COOKIES

1 cup plus 2 tablespoons whole wheat pastry flour
¼ cup teff flour
1 teaspoon baking soda
½ teaspoon salt
1 teaspoon ground cinnamon
¼ teaspoon ground allspice
¼ teaspoon ground cloves
¼ teaspoon ground cardamom

½ cup (1 stick) unsalted butter, at room temperature
¾ cup Sucanat
2 tablespoons blackstrap molasses
½ teaspoon vanilla extract
1 large egg
1 tablespoon freshly grated ginger
⅓ cup white chocolate chips (optional)
⅓ cup dried cranberries (optional)

- Preheat the oven to 350 degrees F. Line two large baking sheets with parchment paper.

- In a medium bowl, whisk together the whole wheat and teff flours, baking soda, salt, cinnamon, allspice, cloves, and cardamom.

- In a large mixing bowl, cream the butter and Sucanat. Add the molasses, vanilla, egg, and ginger and beat until light and fluffy.

- Add flour mixture to the wet ingredients a little at a time. Once incorporated, test the dough to see if you can easily form a ball with moist hands. If the dough sticks, add more whole wheat pastry flour 1 or 2 teaspoons at a time until the dough is soft but pliable and not tacky.

continued

- Form the dough into 1-inch balls with moist hands and place a few inches apart on the baking sheets; they will spread during baking. Dot each dough ball with a chocolate chip or dried cranberry before baking. Bake one sheet at a time for 10 to 12 minutes.

- Let the cookies cool for a few minutes, and then transfer with a spatula to a cooling rack.

PER SERVING (1 cookie): 110 calories, 5 g fat, 1 g protein, 15 g carbohydrates, 1 g fiber, 10 mg sodium

◆ **Chef's Note** ◆

Teff is a sticky grain high in iron that helps lend chewiness to these cookies. The use of iron-rich molasses also helps make them a delicious way to get this important mineral.

Chocolate Chip Cookies

These whole grain cookies contain less fat and sugar than most cookies and make a nutritious snack.

MAKES 30 COOKIES

½ cup (1 stick) butter or no-trans-fat margarine
¼ cup date sugar
¼ cup firmly packed brown sugar
2 egg whites
½ teaspoon vanilla extract
¾ cup whole wheat pastry flour

¼ cup plus 2 tablespoons oat flour
½ teaspoon salt
½ teaspoon baking soda
½ cup nuts (walnuts or pecans are best), chopped
½ cup chocolate chips

• Preheat the oven to 375 degrees F.

• In a mixing bowl, blend the butter and date and brown sugars together until creamy. Beat in the egg whites and vanilla.

• In a separate bowl, sift together the whole wheat and oat flours, salt, and baking soda. Stir into the butter mixture.

• Stir in the nuts and chocolate chips.

• Drop the dough by teaspoonfuls onto a nonstick baking sheet, spacing them several inches apart. Bake for about 10 minutes.

PER SERVING (1 cookie): 71 calories, 4 g fat, 2 g protein, 9 g carbohydrates, 1 g fiber, 70 mg sodium

Very Berry Fruit Crisp

Bursting with the natural sweetness of berries, this "super food" dessert will become a favorite.

MAKES 6 SERVINGS

3 cups fresh or frozen berries (raspberries and marionberries are especially good)

1 to 2 tablespoons cornstarch

¾ cup unbleached all-purpose flour

½ cup rolled oats (regular or quick-cooking)

½ cup nuts (such as pecans, walnuts, almonds, or hazelnuts), chopped

½ cup firmly packed brown sugar

1 teaspoon ground cinnamon

½ teaspoon salt

½ cup (1 stick) butter or no-trans-fat margarine

Vanilla low-fat frozen yogurt

- Preheat the oven to 350 degrees F.

- Place the berries in an 8-inch square baking dish. Mix in 1 tablespoon cornstarch if using fresh berries, or 2 tablespoons if using frozen.

- Combine the flour, oats, nuts, brown sugar, cinnamon, and salt in a mixing bowl. Using clean hands or a fork, work in the butter until the consistency is crumbly. Sprinkle the topping over the berries.

- Bake for 45 minutes, or until golden brown and bubbly. Serve warm, topped with frozen yogurt.

PER SERVING: 388 calories, 22 g fat, 5 g protein, 46 g carbohydrates, 2 g fiber, 335 mg sodium

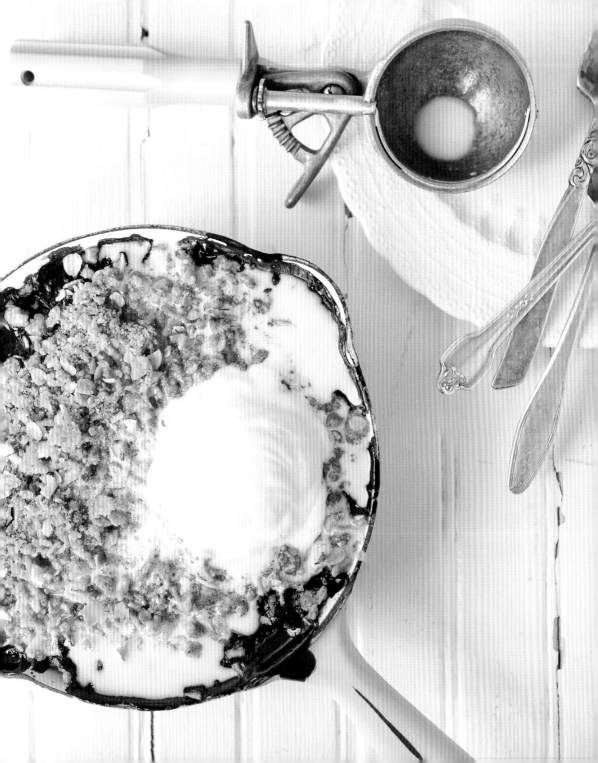

Simply Delicious Berries

Savor the natural sweetness of strawberries in this elegant but simple recipe.

MAKES 4 SERVINGS

1 quart fresh strawberries, rinsed
½ cup powdered sugar

1 cup plain nonfat yogurt

• Arrange the strawberries on a serving plate.

• Set out bowls of the powdered sugar and yogurt for dipping.

PER SERVING: 136 calories, 1 g fat, 4 g protein, 30 g carbohydrates, 2 g fiber, 48 mg sodium

◆ Nutrition Tip ◆

Researchers have found that blueberries, strawberries, and raspberries contain chemicals that help protect against breast and cervical cancer.

Bliss Bars

This easy-to-prepare snack recipe is short in ingredients but long on flavor. Cut into bars, roll into balls, or crumble as a topping over your favorite fresh fruits.

MAKES 6 SERVINGS

½ cup raw almonds

½ cup raw cashews

1 cup dates, pitted

¼ cup raisins

- Pulse the almonds and cashews in a food processor to chop roughly. Add the dates and raisins and process for 1 to 2 minutes, or until a sticky ball forms.

- Lay waxed paper on a cutting board and place the dough in the center.

- Using clean hands, press the dough into a square roughly 6 inches across. Use a flat edge, like a small cutting board or the flat edge of a knife, to square the edges.

- Using a sharp knife, cut into 6 squares or bars. Refrigerate or freeze until serving.

PER SERVING (1 bar): 200 calories, 9 g fat, 5 g protein, 28 g carbohydrates, 4 g fiber, 0 mg sodium

> ♦ Contributor's Note ♦
>
> You can use any kind of nuts (peanuts, walnuts, pecans), and your choice of dried fruit (cherries, cranberries, apples). Coconut, chocolate chips, crystallized ginger, and ground spices are also fun add-ins.

Date Treats

From Sheila Taft, Cancer Lifeline horticultural therapist

Dates have been called nature's candy. Choose either fresh or dried dates that are glossy and plump. Avoid fruit with crystallized sugars on the surface.

MAKES 1 SERVING

5 dates, pitted

5 walnut halves or whole almonds

Shredded coconut or sugar (optional)

- Push the walnuts into center of the dates.

- Sprinkle with shredded coconut. Store in a tightly covered container.

PER SERVING: 209 calories, 10 g fat, 3 g protein, 33 g carbohydrates, 5 g fiber, 3 mg sodium

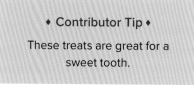

♦ **Contributor Tip** ♦

These treats are great for a sweet tooth.

Baked Custard

A rich, smooth dessert to satisfy your sweet tooth.

MAKES 5 SERVINGS

2 cups reduced-fat milk
¼ to ⅓ cup honey
⅛ teaspoon salt

2 large eggs
1 teaspoon vanilla extract
Ground nutmeg

• Preheat the oven to 325 degrees F. Place 5 custard cups into a baking pan.

• In a medium saucepan over medium-low heat, warm the milk, honey, and salt, stirring until the honey is dissolved.

• In a medium bowl, beat the eggs lightly, then slowly add the warmed milk mixture, whisking constantly. Stir in the vanilla.

• Pour the mixture into the custard cups. Sprinkle with nutmeg. Pour hot water around the cups to a depth of 1 inch.

• Bake for 45 to 60 minutes. The custard is done when a knife blade inserted in the center comes out clean.

PER SERVING: 142 calories, 4 g fat, 6 g protein, 22 g carbohydrates, 0 g fiber, 126 mg sodium

Pumpkin Pie

A full-flavored but low-fat version of a favorite recipe.

MAKES 12 SERVINGS

9 whole graham crackers, finely
   crushed
½ cup fruit juice
4 egg whites, lightly beaten
One 16-ounce can pumpkin
½ cup firmly packed brown sugar

¼ teaspoon salt
1 teaspoon ground cinnamon
½ teaspoon ground ginger
¼ teaspoon ground cloves
One 12-ounce can evaporated
   skim milk

* Preheat the oven to 425 degrees F.

* In a medium bowl, combine the graham cracker crumbs with the fruit juice to moisten. Press into a 9-inch pie pan.

* In a large mixing bowl, combine the egg whites, pumpkin, brown sugar, salt, cinnamon, ginger, cloves, and evaporated milk. Beat until smooth.

* Pour the filling into the prepared pie crust and bake for 15 minutes.

* Reduce the oven temperature to 350 degrees F and bake for an additional 40 to 50 minutes, or until a knife inserted near the center comes out clean. Let cool before serving.

PER SERVING (1 slice): 125 calories, 1 g fat, 4 g protein, 25 g carbohydrates, 1 g fiber, 254 mg sodium

REFERENCES

Introduction

"New science continues to emerge that links . . ." Rock, C.L., et al. (2013). Nutrition and physical activity guidelines for cancer survivors. *CA: A Cancer J Clin*, 62: 242–274.

"The American Cancer Society estimates that nearly one-third of all cancer deaths . . ." American Cancer Society. American Cancer Society Guidelines on Nutrition and Physical Activity for Cancer Prevention. www.cancer.org/acs/groups/cid/documents/webcontent/002577-pdf.pdf.

"In fact, according to cancer experts, if people . . ." American Institute for Cancer Research. (1997). *Food, Nutrition, and the Prevention of Cancer: A Global Perspective*. Washington, DC: American Institute for Cancer Research.

What to Eat and Do Now

"Based on that report and continuous research updates . . ." American Institute for Cancer Research. (1997). *Food, Nutrition, and the Prevention of Cancer: A Global Perspective*. Washington, DC: American Institute for Cancer Research.

American Cancer Society. American Cancer Society Guidelines on Nutrition and Physical Activity for Cancer Prevention. www.cancer.org/acs/groups/cid/documents/webcontent/002577-pdf.pdf.

"Red meat contains heme iron, nitrite, sodium, and compounds . . ." American Institute for Cancer Research. Recommendations for Cancer Prevention. www.aicr.org/reduce-your-cancer-risk/recommendations-for-cancer-prevention/recommendations_05_red_meat.html.

"Research on survivors of cancers . . ." Rock, C.L., et al. (2013). Nutrition and physical activity guidelines for cancer survivors. *CA: A Cancer J Clin*, 62: 242–274.

Top 10 "Super Foods"

"The recommendation for adopting a diet . . ." American Institute for Cancer Research. Phytochemicals: The Cancer Fighters in the Foods We Eat. www.aicr.org/reduce-your-cancer-risk/diet/elements_phytochemicals.html.

"Inflammation is a key player in the production . . ." Cancer Research UK. Feeling the heat—the link between inflammation and cancer. *Science Update*. http://science blog.cancerresearchuk.org/2013/02/01/feeling-the-heat-the-link-between-inflammation-and-cancer.

"A leading researcher on organic foods concluded . . ." The Organic Center. Driving Down Pesticide Risks. www.organic-center.org/reportfiles/DRIfinal11-1[1].pdf.

"According to 43 percent of people . . ." The Organic Center. Do Organic Fruits and Vegetables Taste Better than Conventional Produce. www.organic-center.org/reportfiles/Taste2Pager.pdf.

"These phytochemicals, called glucosinolates . . ." Hayes, J.D., et al. (2008). The cancer chemopreventive actions of phytochemicals derived from glucosinolates. *European Journal of Nutrition*, 47(Suppl 2): 73–88.

"Researchers have found that people who eat more . . ." van Poppel, G., et al. (1999). Brassica vegetables and cancer prevention. Epidemiology and mechanisms, *Adv Exp Med*, 472: 159–68.

"Cancer researchers have determined that protease inhibitors . . ." Gould, M.N. (1997). Cancer chemoprevention and therapy by monoterpenes. *Environ Health Perspect*, 105(Supp 14): 977–79.

"Phytic acid, another beneficial compound . . ." Fox, C.H., & Eberl, M. (2002). Phytic acid (IP6), novel broad spectrum anti-neoplastic agent: a

systematic review. *Complement Ther Med*, 10(4): 229–34.

"The fiber from beans nourish and support friendly bacteria . . ." Tantamango, Y.M., et al. (2011). Foods and food groups associated with the incidence of colorectal polyps: The Adventist health study. *Nutr Cancer*, 63(4): 565–572. doi:10.1080/01635581.2011.551988.

"The ancient Chinese considered soy . . ." Young, V.R., et al. (1984). Evaluation of the protein quality of an isolated soy protein in young men: Relative nitrogen requirements and effect of methionine supplementation. *Am J Clin Nutr*, 39(1): 16–24.

"Soy foods contain phytoestrogens . . ." American Cancer Society. Soybean. www.cancer.org/treatment/treatmentsandsideeffects/complementaryandalternativemedicine/dietandnutrition/soybean.

"If you're a breast cancer survivor . . ." World Cancer Research Fund / American Institute for Cancer Research. (2010). Continuous Update Project Report (summary). Food, Nutrition, Physical Activity, and the Prevention of Breast Cancer. http://www.aicr.org/press/press-releases/soy-safe-breast-cancer-survivors.html.

"A variety of berries and cherries contain powerful antioxidant compounds . . ." Halvorsen, B.L., et al. (2002). A systematic screening of total antioxidants in dietary plants. *J Nutr*, 132: 461–91.

"Anthocyanins in berries may also affect how genes . . ." Stoner, G.D., et al. (2008). Carcinogen-altered genes in rat esophagus positively modulated to normal levels of expression by both black raspberries and phenylethyl isothiocyanate. *Cancer Res*, 68: 6,460–7.

"One researcher identified more than 180 compounds . . ." Benzie I.F., & Wachtel-Gale, S. *Herbal Medicine: Biochemical and Clinical Aspects* (2nd edition). Boca Raton (FL): CRC Press, 2011. Chapter 17: Herbs and Spices in Cancer Prevention and Treatment. www.ncbi.nlm.nih.gov/books/NBK92774/#ch17_sec1.

"Curcumin ranks high in an index of anti-inflammatory foods." Cavicchia, P.P., et al. (2009). A new dietary inflammatory index predicts interval changes in serum high-sensitivity C-reactive protein. *J Nutr*, 139(12): 2,365–72. doi: 10.3945/jn.109.114025.

"In studies of people with a genetic disease . . ." Cruz-Correa, M.C., et al. (2006). Combination treatment with curcumin and quercetin of adenomas in familial adenomatous polyposis. *Clin Gastroenterol Hepatol*, 4(8): 1,035–8. www.ncbi.nlm.nih.gov/pubmed/16757216.

"Ginger may also be helpful an antinausea compound." Benzie, I.F., & Wachtel-Gale, S. *Herbal Medicine: Biochemical and Clinical Aspects* (2nd edition). Boca Raton (FL): CRC Press, 2011. Chapter 17: Herbs and Spices in Cancer Prevention and Treatment. www.ncbi.nlm.nih.gov/books/NBK92774/#ch17_sec1.

"In one study, patients were given . . ." Ryan, J., et al. Ginger (*Zingiber officinale*) reduces acute chemotherapy-induced nausea: a URCC CCOP study of 576 patients. Supportive Care in Cancer. July 2012, Volume 20, Issue 7: pp 1479-1489. http://www.ncbi.nlm.nih.gov/pmc/articles/PMC3361530/.

"Garlic is rich in sulfur . . ." Benzie, I.F., & Wachtel-Gale, S. *Herbal Medicine: Biochemical and Clinical Aspects* (2nd edition). Boca Raton (FL): CRC Press, 2011. http://www.ncbi.nlm.nih.gov/books/NBK92774/#ch17_sec1.

"Human studies on the action of garlic on cancer. . ." American Institute for Cancer Research. Foods That Fight Cancer. www.aicr.org/foods-that-fight-cancer/foodsthatfightcancer_garlic.html.

"A number of fruits and vegetables contain compounds called carotenoids . . ." Craig, W.J. (1997). Phytochemicals: guardians of our health. *J Am Diet Assoc*, 97(10 Suppl 2): S199–204.

"Fish is rich in omega-3 fatty acids . . ." Fernandez, E., et al. (1999). Fish consumption and cancer risk. *Am J Clin Nutr*, 70(1): 85–90.

"Fish seems to protect against cancer . . ." Reddy, B.S., et al. (1991). Effect of diets high in omega-3 and omega-6 fatty acids on initiation and postinitiation stages of colon carcinogenesis. *Cancer Res*, 51: 487–91.

"Research scientists found that DHA . . ." Science Daily. Omega-3 Kills Cancer Cells. www.sciencedaily.com/releases/2009/04/090401200441.htm

"Tomatoes contain lycopene . . ." Heber, D., & Lu, Q.Y. (2002). Overview of mechanisms of action of lycopene. *Exp Biol Med*, 227(10): 920–23.

"This phytonutrient also helps to restore . . ." Bertram, J.S. (1999). Carotenoids and gene regulation. *Nur Rev*, 57(6): 182–91.

"One study showed that when men ate . . ." Giovannucci, E., et al. (1995). Intake of carotenoids and retinol in relation to risk of prostate cancer. *J Natl Cancer Inst*, 87: 1,767–76.

"Mushrooms have been revered in . . . ," "Other mushrooms, including shiitake and maitake . . . ," and "Shiitake mushrooms contain a form of . . ." Ng, M.L., & Yap, A.T. (2002). Inhibition of human colon carcinoma development by lentinan from shiitake mushrooms (*Lentinus edodes*). *J Altern Complement Med*, 8(5): 581–89.

"White button mushrooms, readily available and less costly . . ." Grube, B.J., et al. (2001). White button mushroom phytochemicals inhibit aromatase activity and breast cancer cell proliferation. *J Nutr*. 131(12): 3,288–93.

"The maitake mushroom, also known as . . ." Kodama, N., et al. (2002). Effects of D-fraction, a polysaccharide from *Grifola frondosa* on tumor growth involve activation of NK cells. *Biol Pharm Bull*, 25(12): 1,647–50.

"Nuts appear to have a positive effect on . . ." Hebert, J.R., et al. (1998). Nutritional and socioeconomic factors in relation to prostate cancer mortality: a cross-national study. *J Natl Cancer Inst*, 90(21): 1,637–47.

"In animal studies, walnuts slowed the growth of colon cancer . . ." Nagel, J.M., et al. (2012). Dietary walnuts inhibit colorectal cancer growth in mice by suppressing angiogenesis. *Nutrition*, 28(1): 67–75. doi: 10.1016/j.nut.2011.03.004.

"In another study, mice who were engineered to develop . . ." Davis, P.A., et al. (2012). A high-fat diet containing whole walnuts (*Juglans regia*) reduces tumour size and growth along with plasma insulin-like growth factor 1 in the transgenic adenocarcinoma of the mouse prostate model. *Br J Nutr*, 108(10): 1,764–72. doi: 10.1017/S0007114511007288.

"Lignans in flaxseed protected mice exposed to radiation . . ." Christofidou-Solomidou, M., et al. (2011). Dietary flaxseed administered post thoracic radiation treatment improves survival and mitigates radiation-induced pneumonopathy in mice. *BMC Cancer*.

"Flaxseed (30 grams a day) and a low-fat diet (20 percent fat) lowered . . ." American Institute for Cancer Research. (2002). *Nutrition After Cancer*, 20–26. Washington DC: American Institute for Cancer Research.

"In animal studies, flaxseed did not interfere with tamoxifen's actions . . ." American Institute for Cancer Research. AICR InDepth. Flaxseeds and Breast Cancer by Karen Collins, MS, RD, CDN. http://www.aicr.org/assets/docs/pdf/education/FlaxseedBreastCancer.pdf.

"Polyphenols in tea are known to inhibit . . ." Kazi, A., et al. (2002). Potential molecular targets of tea polyphenols in human tumor cells: significance in cancer prevention. *In Vivo*, 16(6): 397–403.

"Researchers who reviewed population studies found that . . ." Ogunleye, A.A., et al. (2010). Green tea consumption and breast cancer risk or recurrence: a meta-analysis. *Breast Cancer Res Treat*, 119(2): 477–84. doi: 10.1007/s10549-009-0415-0.

"Men with prostate cancer who drank six cups of green tea . . ." Science Daily. Green Tea Reduced Inflammation, May Inhibit Prostate Cancer Tumor Growth. www.sciencedaily.com/releases/2012/10/121018121956.htm.

Nutrients That Promote Good Health

"Eating large quantities of red meat . . ." National Cancer Institute. Animal Foods by Arthur Schatzkin, M.D., Dr.P.H. www.dietandcancerreport.org/cancer_resource_center/downloads/speaker_slides/us/06_Schatzkin_Animal_Foods.pdf.

"Although all types of fat have similar amounts of calories . . ." and Types of Fat. Harvard School of Public Health. Fats and Cholesterol: Out with the Bad, In with the Good. www.hsph.harvard.edu/nutritionsource/fats-full-story.

"Researchers found that the men with nonmetastatic prostate cancer . . ." Richman, E.L., et al. (2013). Fat Intake After Diagnosis and Risk of Lethal Prostate Cancer and All-Cause Mortality. *JAMA Intern Med*.

"The recommended intake of omega-3 fatty acids . . ." Gebauer, S.K., et.al. (2006). n-3 fatty acid dietary recommendations and food sources to achieve essentiality and cardiovascular benefits. *Am J Clin Nutr*, 83(6 Suppl): 1,526S–1,535S.

"But when they're consumed in popular processed foods . . ." ChooseMyPlate.gov. What Are Empty Calories. www.choosemyplate.gov/weight-management-calories/calories/empty-calories.html.

"Hydrogenated fats (also called trans fats) . . ." and "Hydrogenated fats should be avoided . . ." Mayo Clinic. Trans Fat Is Double Trouble for Your Heart Health. www.mayoclinic.com/health/trans-fat/CL00032.

"Diets rich in foods containing . . ." American Cancer Society. Calcium. www.cancer.org/treatment/treatmentsandsideeffects/complementaryandalternativemedicine/herbsvitaminsandminerals/calcium.

"Several studies have suggested that foods high in calcium . . ." American Cancer Society. Calcium. www.cancer.org/treatment/treatmentsandsideeffects/complementaryandalternativemedicine/herbsvitaminsandminerals/calcium.

"Researchers found that men who had higher levels . . ." American Association for Cancer Research. Cohort Study Indicates That Selenium May Be Protective Against Advanced Prostate Cancer. www.aacr.org/home/public—media/aacr-in-the-news.aspx?d=3058.

"Sea vegetables contain ten to twenty times . . ." Bradford, P., & Bradford, M. (1988). *Cooking with Sea Vegetables*, 10–15. Rochester, VT: Healing Arts Press.

Creating a Healthier Diet

"In a primarily plant-based diet . . ." American Institute for Cancer Research. (1997). *Food, Nutrition, and the Prevention of Cancer: A Global Perspective*, 14–15. Washington, D.C: American Institute for Cancer Research.

"In the United States, excess body weight . . ." American Cancer Society. Does Body Weight Affect Cancer Risk? www.cancer.org/cancer/cancercauses/dietandphysicalactivity/bodyweightandcancerrisk/body-weight-and-cancer-risk-effects.

"In one study, researchers gathered information . . ." American Institute for Cancer Research. Study: Cutting Premature Death with AICR Recommendations. www.aicr.org/cancer-research-update/april_03_2013/cru_cutting_premature_death.html.

"If you are obese or overweight, modest weight loss . . ." Rock, C.L., et al. (2013). Nutrition and physical activity guidelines for cancer survivors. *CA: A Cancer J Clin*, 62: 242–274.

"The ACS offers general guidelines on food safety . . ." Rock C.L., et al. (2013). Nutrition and physical activity guidelines for cancer survivors. *CA: A Cancer J Clin*, 62: 242–274.

"Avoid eating alfalfa sprouts . . ." US Department of Health and Human Services, Food and Drug Administration. (1999). Consumers Advised of Risks Associated with Raw Sprouts. www.cfsan.fda.gov/~lrd/hhssprts.html.

"Certain types of plastic . . ." Singleton, D.W., & Khan, S.A. (2003). Xenoestrogen exposure and mechanisms of endocrine disruption. *Front Biosci*, 8: S110–18.

"Animal foods, such as red meat . . ." American Institute for Cancer Research. Cancer Experts Offer Seasonal Advice for Safer Grilling. www.aicr.org/enews/2012/june-2012/enews-cancer-experts-offer.html.

Coping with Possible Side Effects of Cancer Treatment

"Ginger (*Zingiber officinalis*) is an herb recognized . . ." Duke, J. (1997). *The Green Pharmacy*, 410. New York: St. Martin's Press.

Watermelon Popsicle recipe. Warren, J. (1992). *Super Snacks*, 43. Torrance, CA: Frank Schaeffer Publications.

Try Honey for a Sore Throat. Maiti, P.K., et al. (2012). The effect of honey on mucositis induced by chemoradiation in head and neck cancer. *J Indian Med Assoc*, 110(7): 453–6.

FASS for Taste Changes. Caring4Cancer. Finding Comfort, Joy, and Healing in Food. www.caring4cancer.com/go/cancer/nutrition/chef-rebecca-katz.

Getting Organized

Should You Buy Organic? Chensheng, L., et al. (2006). Organic diets significantly lower children's dietary exposure to organophosphorus pesticides. *Environmental Health Perspectives*. www.ncbi.nlm.nih.gov/pmc/articles/PMC1367841.

"Organic meat and poultry means . . ." Center for Science in the Public Interest. Nutrition Action Healthletter. (2012). www.cspinet.org.

"Experts recommend limiting added sugars . . ." American Heart Association. Sugars and Carbohydrates. www.heart.org/HEARTORG/GettingHealthy/NutritionCenter/HealthyDietGoals/Sugars-and-Carbohydrates_UCM_303296_Article.jsp.

Ideas for Quick-Fix Meals. American Dietetic Association. Vegetarian Nutrition Dietetic Practice Group. (2001). *Quick Vegetarian Meals*. Chicago, IL: American Dietetic Assoc.

Ideas for Quick-Fix Meals. American Institute for Cancer Research. (1994). *Healthy Meals on Hand*. Washington, DC: American Institute for Cancer Research.

Ideas for Quick-Fix Meals. Warren, J. (1992). *Super Snacks*. Torrance, CA: Frank Schaeffer Publications.

GLOSSARY

ALLYL SULFIDES AND DIALLYL DISULFIDES (DADS): Sulfur-containing compounds found in vegetables of the onion family that act as cancer-blocking or cancer-suppressing agents.

ALPHA-LINOLENIC ACID: Fatty acid of the omega-3 type.

ANTHOCYANINS: Plant-based chemicals that give blue, blue-red, and purple colors to berries. These compounds act as antioxidants.

ANTIOXIDANTS: Any of a variety of naturally occurring substances—such as vitamins A, E, and C; beta-carotene; and selenium—that can prevent or impede oxidation reactions.

BETA-GLUCAN (D-FRACTION): Compounds found in maitake mushrooms that may stimulate the immune system and activate certain cells and proteins that attack cancer.

CARCINOGENS: Cancer-causing substances.

CAROTENOIDS: A class of plant pigments found in dark green and orange vegetables and fruits that have proven antioxidant and immune-regulatory abilities.

CRUCIFEROUS VEGETABLES: A group of vegetables (including cauliflower, cabbage, brussels sprouts, broccoli, turnips, and rutabagas) containing substances that may protect against and fight cancer.

DETOXIFICATION ENZYMES: Liver enzymes that transform toxic molecules into water-soluble compounds that can be eliminated from the body.

ELLAGIC ACID: A plant-based chemical found in walnuts that may slow cancer cell growth. Also beneficial in lowering high blood cholesterol levels.

ENZYMES: Proteinlike substances formed in plant and animal cells that act as catalysts in initiating or speeding up specific chemical reactions. Usually destroyed by high temperatures.

FLAVONOIDS: A group of plant pigments proven to protect against free-radical damage. They are noted for their anti-inflammatory, antiviral, antiallergenic, and anticancer activities.

FREE RADICALS: Highly reactive compounds with at least one unpaired electron, formed naturally within the body as a result of metabolic processes. The body is also exposed to free radicals as a result of sun exposure (radiation), smoking, drug and alcohol use, pollution, and stress. Free radicals can cause oxidative damage to cell membranes, tissue, and DNA, and contribute to aging and disease progression, including cancer.

HETEROCYCLIC AMINES (HCA): Cancer-causing compounds formed when animal foods are barbecued, cooked on hot stones, fried, or broiled.

HYDROGENATED FAT: Polyunsaturated fats that have been chemically changed. These fats are widely used by the food industry in prepared foods, deep-fried foods, and shortenings. Like saturated fats, hydrogenated fats have a negative health impact.

INDOLES: A group of compounds found in cruciferous vegetables that have exhibited anticancer activity.

ISOFLAVONE: A group of compounds found in soy and other plant foods that may block the entry of estrogen into cells, reducing the risk of breast and ovarian cancer.

LACTOSE: A form of sugar found in milk and other dairy products.

LACTOSE INTOLERANCE: The inability to digest milk sugar (lactose) due to insufficient production of lactase, the enzyme that digests lactose. Lactase production typically declines with age and may be reduced by certain diseases and disease treatments that cause changes to the small intestine.

LEGUMES: The protein-rich seeds of plants such as kidney beans, soybeans, garden peas, lentils, black-eyed peas, and lima beans. Legumes are a good source of soluble fiber and can exert a stabilizing effect on blood sugar levels.

LENTINAN: A form of complex sugar molecule in mushrooms that may stimulate the immune system and provide anticancer protection.

LIGNAN: Compounds found in flaxseed that are transformed by the bacteria in our bodies into hormonelike substances (phytoestrogens) that may protect against tumor formation and growth.

LYCOPENE: A plant-based chemical found in tomatoes, watermelon, and other red and pink fruits and vegetables. Lycopene appears to reduce the risk of prostate and breast cancer.

MACRONUTRIENTS: Protein, carbohydrates, and fats. They are called macronutrients because the body needs them in large quantities.

MACROPHAGE: A type of white blood cell that filters the lymph system, engulfing foreign particles such as bacteria and cellular debris.

MICRONUTRIENTS: Vitamins and minerals. They are called micronutrients because the body needs them in small quantities.

MONOUNSATURATED FATS: These fats, which are liquid at room temperature, come from plant sources that include olive, canola, avocado, and nuts and seeds—like pumpkin seeds, walnuts, and peanuts. They help to protect heart health.

MUCILAGE: A soft, moist, and viscous compound secreted by the seed covers of various plants, such as flax and slippery elm.

NITROSAMINES: Carcinogens formed during digestion from nitrites—food additives used to prevent bacterial growth in processed meats such as hot dogs, bacon, ham, and sausage. In adequate doses, vitamin C can prevent the transformation of nitrites into nitrosamines.

OMEGA-3 POLYUNSATURATED FATTY ACIDS: Fats found in cold-water fish, such as salmon, mackerel, and herring, and in certain plants, nuts, and seeds, such as walnuts, flaxseed, and pumpkin seeds. Omega-3 fatty acids have been shown to positively affect immune responses, reduce the inflammation response to injury and infection, decrease the formation of blood clots, lower blood pressure, and reduce cholesterol.

OMEGA-6 POLYUNSATURATED FATS: Highly polyunsaturated fatty acids found primarily in animal proteins and vegetable oils. Modern diets are more abundant in this fatty acid than in omega-3 fatty acids.

PHYTIC ACID: A phosphorous-containing compound found principally in the outer husks of cereal grains.

PHYTOCHEMICALS: "Phyto-" means plant. "Phytochemicals" is a generalized term for a wide group of naturally occurring substances, such as carotenoids, that are found in plants and have been shown to have anticancer effects.

PHYTOESTROGENS: Natural substances, found in soy and other plant foods, that exert estrogenlike effects. Compared to estrogen, phytoestrogen's activity is only 1:100,000. Because of this weak effect, phytoestrogens tend to counteract extreme estrogen levels. If estrogen levels are low, they will cause an increase in estrogen effect. If levels are too high, phytoestrogens will bind to estrogen-binding sites, thus decreasing estrogen's effects. In men, phytoestrogens seem to block testosterone, the hormone that can spur the growth of prostate tumors.

PHYTOSTEROLS: Substances found in plants that may slow the production of cells in the large intestine and therefore slow tumor growth.

POLYPHENOLS: An antioxidative group of phytochemicals.

POLYSACCHARIDE: A large and complex molecule made up of smaller sugar molecules.

PROSTAGLANDINS: Modified fatty acids that act in the body as messengers involved in reproduction and the inflammatory response to infection.

PROTEASE INHIBITORS: Compounds that inhibit the action of protein-digesting enzymes and may retard the growth of human colon and breast cancer cells.

POLYCYCLIC AROMATIC HYDROCARBONS (PAHS): Cancer-causing compounds formed when fat drips from grilled or broiled animal foods onto hot coals or stones. Smoke and flare-ups deposit these compounds on foods.

POLYSACCHARIDE: A form of highly complex carbohydrates found in plants.

PSYLLIUM: A soluble fiber that comes from a plant most commonly grown in India. Soluble fiber aids in intestinal health and regularity.

SAPONIN: A sugar compound with emulsifying properties. Saponins are thought to interfere with the process by which DNA replicates and may prevent cancer cells from multiplying.

SELENIUM: A trace mineral and important antioxidant that may help prevent cancer formation and promotion. Selenium functions either alone or as part of enzyme systems. Although selenium is needed only in small amounts, insufficient intake is common because of selenium-deficient soils. Low-selenium diets have been associated with an increased risk of cancer.

SULPHORAPHANE: A sulfur-based chemical found in plants that may stimulate enzymes in the body to destroy cancer-causing agents.

T-LYMPHOCYTE: A form of white blood cell that recognizes and reacts to parasites, cancer cells, and cells infected by viruses.

INDEX

Note: Photographs are indicated by *italics*.

A

appetite, loss of, 55–56, 58
appetizers and salads, 101–119
apples
    Apple Muesli, 90
    Pecan-Honey-Baked
        Apples, 214
    Raisin-Apple-Date
        Cookies, 215
    Waldorf Salad, 110, *111*
Artichoke Dip, Creamy, 117
Arugula, Spelt Pilaf with
    Baby, 164
Asparagus-Mushroom Stir-Fry
    with Bay Scallops, 189
Avocado-Dressed Fresh Kale
    Salad, 107
Avocado Soup, Chilled, 134,
    135

B

Banana Bran Muffins, 93
Bars, Bliss, 223
beans, 6, *13*, 14–16, 30, 31,
    36, 40
    Black Bean Soup, 132
    Black-Eyed Pea and Ham
        Soup, 125
    Breakfast Burritos, 92
    Creamy Polenta and Bean
        Casserole, 197

Honey-Glazed Green
    Beans with Almonds,
    147
Lickety-Split Hummus, 118
Roasted Beets and Beet
    Greens with Marcona
    Almonds and Zolfini
    Beans, 151–152, *153*
Spicy Chickpea, Kale, and
    Tomato Stew, 200–201
Stovetop Fish Stew with
    Gingered Black Beans,
    174
Texas Black Bean Salad,
    108
Three-Bean Vegetarian
    Chili, 205
Beet and Yogurt Soup, Masala,
    124
Beets and Beet Greens with
    Marcona Almonds and
    Zolfini Beans, Roasted,
    151–152, *153*
berries, 16–17, 35, 36, 51, 52
    Blueberry Breakfast Cake,
        94, 95
    Great Grains Breakfast
        Cereal, *88*, 89
    Simply Delicious Berries,
        222
    Tropical Salsa, 119
    Very Berry Fruit Crisp,
        220, *221*
    Yogurt Protein Shake,
        86–87

Bouillabaisse, Seattle, 172, *173*
Bran Muffins, Banana, 93
Bread, Quick Corn, 155
Bread, Roasted Garlic, 156
breakfast, 85–100
broccoli, 29, 33, 35, 36
    Broccoli and Lamb Stir-Fry
        with Soy-Sherry Sauce,
        193–194
    Broccoli with Sesame-
        Crusted Tofu, 148
    "Cream" of Broccoli Soup,
        129
    Crunchy Broccoli and
        Carrot Salad, 105
    Curried Root Vegetables,
        138, 139
    Pork Yakisoba, 190, *191*
buckwheat, 157, 160
Burritos, Breakfast, 92

C

calcium, 35–36, 37
Cancer Lifeline, 3–4, 62
cancer treatment, side effects
    of, 18, 27–29, 30, 31, 35, 37,
    42–43, 47–60
carbohydrates, 31, 71
carotenoids, *13*, 19–20, 24,
    234
Carrot Salad, Crunchy
    Broccoli and, 105
Carrot Soup, Gingered, 136
Casserole, Creamy Polenta and
    Bean, 197

239

ACKNOWLEDGMENTS

CANCER LIFELINE OWES A LARGE DEBT OF GRATITUDE TO THE MANY individuals whose expertise, effort, and enthusiasm helped us bring this version of the cookbook to press. Thank you to Kimberly Mathai, MS, RD, CDE, who devoted her time and energy in writing and researching this new edition. We gratefully acknowledge Julie Hillers, Cancer Lifeline board member, and program director Joseph Yurgavitch. Julie provided invaluable technical advice and shared her love of all things cooking; Joseph made the project a reality with his enthusiasm and encouragement. Gary Luke, President at Sasquatch Books, provided us the opportunity to bring this latest edition to press.

We would also like to extend special thanks to Rachel Keim—author of the first edition—and Ginny Smith, who edited both the first and second editions; and the staff at both Cancer Lifeline and Sasquatch Books. Their professional expertise, talent, and dedication have played a major role in bringing this book to fruition.

To those who contributed recipes and tips to this current edition, we are grateful for your insight and culinary talent. Mary Mataja, Julie Hillers, Cynthia Lair, Jerry Traunfeld, and Bharti Kirchner for contributing new recipes to this version of the cookbook. We reiterate our thanks to the many people who contributed to previous editions of the cookbook. A big thanks goes to volunteers Sarah Beyler, Rachel Bishop, Justin Daigneault, Nancy Miller, and Annbritah Kabiru, who all tested and analyzed recipes. At the time of this writing, all were students in the Department of Nutrition and Dietetics at Bastyr University in Seattle, Washington.

ABOUT THE AUTHOR

KIMBERLY MATHAI, MS, RD, CDE, is a registered dietitian and certified diabetes educator. She is the nutrition educator at Cancer Lifeline, a nonprofit support center for people with cancer and their caregivers. She has a private nutrition consulting practice with Your Nutrition Design (YourNutritionDesign.com), in Seattle. Mathai has written extensively on nutrition for medical textbooks, Internet-based companies, and popular magazines. She received her master's degree in nutrition from Seattle's Bastyr University.